CW00456720

# Nurturing Yourself Through IVF

# Nurturing Yourself Through IVF

## Improve Your Experience
## Maximize Your Odds of Success

Lynn Daley

LIFE PRINTS

NOTE: *This book is not designed to take the place of medical care. Please consult your physician or reproductive endocrinologist with any questions regarding your physical care.*

*If you choose to follow the principles of Traditional Chinese Medicine, be sure to consult with trained professionals: licensed acupuncturists or doctors of Oriental medicine. Let your reproductive endocrinologist know that you are supplementing treatment with alternative therapies.*

*Please note that the names of the women quoted in this book have been changed to protect their privacy.*

Copyright © 2006 Life Prints.

First Edition

All rights reserved. No part of this book may be reproduced in any form or by any electronic or mechanical means, including information storage and retrieval systems, without written permission of the publisher, except by a reviewer who may quote brief passages in a review.

**Library and Archives Canada Cataloguing in Publication**

Daley, Lynn, 1971–

Nurturing yourself through IVF : improve your experience, maximize your odds of success / Lynn Daley.

Includes bibliographical references.

ISBN 0-9739860-0-X

1. Fertilization in vitro, Human—Popular works.  2. Women—Health and hygiene.  I. Title.

RG135.D345 2006          618.1'780599          C2006-901062-5

Cover image courtesy of Atmospheric Optics:
http://www.atoptics.co.uk

Dedicated to the women I've met
in waiting rooms, on trains, at work,
through friends, over the phone and online.
May you be blessed with healthy children,
and may your generosity of spirit
reward you throughout your lives.

May all reading this book
find the peace of mind
and the sense of being 'whole'
that you so deserve.

To my wonderful husband,
thank you.

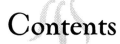

# Contents

1.  Introduction: A New Way to View IVF ...................................1

2.  An Important Understanding ...................................7

3.  Am I *Really* Meant to Experience This?...................................13

4.  Understanding Your Energy...................................28

5.  Embracing Your Natural Advantage...................................33

6.  Being Kind To Yourself...................................41

7.  Finding Your Life Raft ...................................48

8.  Editing The World Around You ...................................60

9.  Creating Your New To-Do List...................................75

10. You Can Do This...................................88

11. Conclusion...................................92

    Appendix One: A Few Great Resources...................................94

    Appendix Two: One Successful Cycle...................................104

# Chapter One

# Introduction:
# A New Way to View IVF

So OFTEN, A GREAT ENDING has a difficult beginning. If your journey to parenthood includes In-Vitro Fertilization (IVF), chances are good that your beginning has already been full of challenge.

You may wonder if you'll ever get to your happy ending. You will likely ask yourself how you landed on this bumpy, unpleasant road toward something that seems so easy for almost everyone else.

Going through IVF is much more than a logical step in a couple's journey to parenthood. It is an emotional leap of faith, a time of truth when a couple is challenged in ways that they might not have imagined possible.

Women, who naturally shoulder most of the effort involved in IVF, usually find the experience taxing on their emotions, on their bodies, and on their ability to function normally in their lives outside of fertility treatments.

If you are a woman going through IVF, if you are between cycles, or if you suspect that IVF may be part of your future, this book has been written for you. It has been designed to help you learn to put yourself first, which is not something that comes easily to most women. Ultimately, I hope that you are able to view your entire IVF experience from a healthy, new perspective.

As you learn specific ways to improve your experience, you will naturally improve your state of mind and the conditions of your physical body. This connection between your mind and body is important and enormously powerful. It just might provide you with the advantage that you need to achieve a successful pregnancy.

Nurturing yourself through IVF is about giving yourself the time and permission to put yourself first. It is about getting to and through your cycle with a sense of calm, positive energy. It is about upholding your sense of self with the utmost respect and esteem. Finally, it is about 'getting back to yourself' and trusting that no matter how your journey unfolds, that you will be okay.

## Beyond the Numbers

Because IVF is a medical procedure, it is very easy to fall into a clinical mindset. Each fertility clinic will be able to recite your chances of success per cycle. Your carefully-measured drugs will have a target number of eggs produced. Embryos are closely observed so that they can be assessed and graded. It can all seem very black and white.

The medical component of IVF can be so overwhelming that it is easy to put aside the other major component in a cycle: *you*. How will you feel through the cycle? How will that affect your outcome? How can you maximize your odds of success by using the natural healing powers of your mind?

In order to make the most of the material presented in this book, it is important for you to keep an open mind. We will cover concepts that may seem somewhat abstract when you have grown used to a mindset of scientific procedures and statistical odds.

Once you understand how your feelings affect your energy and your physical conditions, you can work to make simple changes in your daily life that not only feel good, but will also help to improve your odds of success. Happily, these changes can also provide you with a greater sense of control and self-confidence.

## A Sense of Hope

Throughout the following chapters, I will share my own experiences, as well as those of some of the women that I have met along the way. The intent is not to make this book about me or anyone else, but rather to share information and feelings that may help you through your own IVF journey.

I wrote this book because I felt that there was something missing in literature surrounding IVF. Recently, some terrific resources have emerged that address alternative therapies or approaches to infertility. I thought there needed to be something that addressed IVF specifically, however, and that it needed to be written by someone who had been through it.

My own experience includes three IVF cycles: two fresh and one frozen. Over the course of the three years that it took to achieve a successful pregnancy, I did plenty of reading and spoke to over one hundred women going through IVF.

Although I was receiving excellent medical care, I knew that I needed more. I desperately needed to feel that I could do something to improve my odds of success. I needed to fuel a sense of hope with deliberate action.

As I searched for ways that I could improve my odds, I began to take an interest in learning how my feelings and energy could help me to improve my physical conditions. Herein lay a set of tools that allowed me to preserve my hope and to foster a belief that things would somehow work out.

Through my own experience and subsequent research, I've heard stories of heart-felt frustration and sorrow, as well as those of hope and inspiration. I've learned about current tests and procedures, about new research, and perhaps most important, about the impact that IVF can have on a woman's sense of self.

I am not a doctor, nor a certified expert in psychology, nutrition or natural healing therapies. What I do have, is extensive experience in speaking with women going through IVF, a willingness to share what worked for me and a belief that you too can maximize your odds of success with an open mind and heart.

## Simple Goals

As you read this book, I have three simple goals for you:

### i) For you to feel connected

I hope that you see events, circumstances and emotions that strike you as familiar. The women quoted throughout this book were at very different stages of their cycles, and had very different circumstances from one another. I hope that you are able to see yourself in some of these stories.

## ii) For you to embrace simple tools and techniques

Throughout this book, you will find tools that help you to keep a calm sense of perseverance through your IVF journey. They focus on making you feel better, which should come as a relief for your battered emotions. Given the right opportunity, these techniques can change the way you experience your fertility journey altogether. I hope that you are able to give them an honest chance.

## iii) To motivate you to pursue your own research

As you will see, I researched plenty of routes and theories on my road to IVF success. What ultimately worked for me, however, may not be your style or your best route to success. I hope that this book provides you with the motivation to pursue your own best path.

## Moving Forward

I truly believe that even though you may have been meant to experience IVF, you were also meant to get through it with the best possible outcome. As with any challenge, you will best be prepared to succeed if you are able to keep an open mind to new solutions and are willing to trust your instinct.

If this is your first time going through IVF, you may feel overwhelmed by the emotions and physical demands of the cycle. I hope that you will find comfort in learning that you are not alone.

If you have been through IVF at least once, you may be somewhat skeptical out of self-defense. I hope that this book offers you a fresh perspective and some new ideas to help maximize your odds of success.

I wish you more than luck on your journey ahead. I wish you peace of mind, a healthy body and firm focus on your goal of having a baby. More than anything, I hope that you can nurture a sense of faith that no matter how things unfold, you will be okay.

# CHAPTER TWO
# An Important Understanding

LIKE MANY OF LIFE'S STRUGGLES, it is nearly impossible for people who haven't experienced IVF to truly know what it is like. This is not to say that a friend or family member can't be a great source of support, it's just that he or she can't truly understand all that you're going through.

There are too many difficult situations to explain, too many days when you wake up wondering if it will ever happen, and often too many disappointments to try and express all of your feelings to someone who hasn't been there.

As women who *can* understand the logistics and emotions of a fertility struggle, it is very important that we share our support with one another. Together, we have an understanding. We have a likeness and an underlying sense of empathy for one another.

Connecting with other women has another important benefit: it allows you to share and receive valuable information that can improve your odds of success. Because the research behind IVF is steadily evolving, it is important to share as much information

ːible. Information passed on from one woman's doctor or experience may eventually help another to find success.

## Dueling Emotions

My personal journey through IVF took many bumps and turns. Like the vast majority of couples going through this process, my husband Paul and I had gone through many months of waiting, tests and disappointment before considering advanced treatment. The journey was filled with highs and lows, and had taken its toll on both of us.

After a long wait to get in to see our Reproductive Endocrinologist (RE), we began a heightened pattern of hope and fear. Upon his recommendation, Paul had surgery to remove a varicocele (enlarged veins in the scrotum), in hopes that it would improve his sperm count and quality. I also underwent laparoscopic surgery to see whether or not I had endometriosis.

The results were disappointing. Paul's sperm count only improved marginally. Although my surgery revealed only a mild case of endometriosis, our RE still considered this significant; he worried that it may affect my fertility at a microscopic level.

As time marched on and more test results came in, we were starting to feel that the odds were stacked against us. Fortunately, IVF offered a tremendous amount of new hope. I felt relieved and optimistic as our cycle drew near.

As things progressed, however, my optimism was suddenly challenged by complete and utter fear. What if, despite our extensive efforts and expensive treatment, it still didn't work? I was sure that I couldn't handle that sort of disappointment.

When my pregnancy test came back negative, my biggest fears had materialized. Now, instead of wondering if I could handle the disappointment, I had to find a place for it. I was surprised by the power and intensity of these feelings.

More than anything, I wanted to be alone. I didn't want anyone's consolation, not even my husband's. I didn't think that anyone could truly understand how devastated I felt. All that I wanted was to find an escape, from my social life, from work, from everything.

## Finding Support

At the time of that first cycle, I didn't know anyone else going through IVF. Although I saw plenty of women at the clinic each morning, it didn't feel like the right environment to form friendships.

Naturally, we were all tired and worried. Some faces looked mad, others just weary. None of us wanted to be there. Despite my physical proximity to these other women, I felt quite alone.

Fortunately, it wasn't long after that first cycle that I decided to look online for some sense of hope. I stumbled across a bulletin board site called IVF Connections, where I met a group of women who knew *just* how I felt. Their support was both emotional and practical; they helped me to feel connected, understood and better about myself.

Soon thereafter, I began to explore other online support groups, as well. They offered an anonymous, comforting setting where I could learn, vent, and explore. I was surprised that I could feel so connected, so quickly.

One of the women that I met during this time was Holly. She was just heading into her second cycle, and was remembering her feelings from her first experience.

> I was so surprised how hard it was to keep my
> spirits up. It was like I couldn't let myself feel
> excitement at any stage without immediately
> feeling doubt. I was going straight from hope
> into tears...I just felt out of control.
>
> —HOLLY, 32

By sharing experiences, feelings and information with women like Holly, I could feel that my attitude towards IVF was beginning to change. Although my disappointment remained very real, I became more determined, more resolute and more positive. Thankfully, this was true even as things got worse.

## A Pragmatic Turn

Over the next 10 months, under the direction of our RE and through our own initiative, we began to look high and low for possible routes to success. Our RE suggested that I undergo a new diagnostic test called the Endometrial Function Test, followed by two months of a drug called Depot Lupron. Two months later, I racked up another IVF failure through a frozen transfer. Things weren't looking up.

Between these two first cycles, Paul and I consulted with four clinics and six doctors. I sent my blood out of country for specialized, expensive testing. In an effort to support these tactics, I had also begun to explore the benefits of Traditional Chinese Medicine (TCM), acupuncture and basic relaxation techniques.

Although there was little scientific proof that these alternative therapies would help in my situation, I knew that I needed to *do something* to feel more proactive. I wanted no stone unturned; if we did eventually move on to surrogacy or adoption, I wanted to know that we had done everything possible to carry and have our own biological child.

## A Better Experience

Ultimately, I was able to renew my view of IVF and its role in my life. With the help of some of the techniques that we will cover in this book, I learned how to handle setbacks and waiting periods with a greater sense of purpose and calm. As I learned to 'let go' and level out my personal energy, I felt a sense of control come flooding back into my life.

After several months, in combination with my IVF procedures, treatment for my immune system and supplemental therapies (diet, relaxation and acupuncture), I was able to achieve a successful pregnancy. I have many people to thank for their assistance.

I need to thank my doctors for their skilled treatment. I also have many women to thank for their information, motivation and support. Without their help, I would not have known where to seek immune system testing, I wouldn't have learned about relaxation techniques, nor would I have explored the benefits of acupuncture or Chinese medicine.

They also offered an emotional understanding that improved my experience altogether. I am entirely grateful for the generosity and good will of the women that I have met.

## Your Own Direction

In "Appendix Two: One Successful Cycle," I list all of the things that we did in the cycle that worked for us. The only reason I do so is that I know exactly how you feel about reading a book on IVF—you want to know what *works*, and what you might be able to do to improve your odds of success.

I should make it clear, however, that in no way do I want to suggest that you follow my exact course of action to achieve your own pregnancy. Even if you share my diagnosis and circumstances, my direction may not be the answer for you. Given the information that I had at the time, it just turned out to be the best answer for me.

What I do recommend, however, is that you embrace the very idea that you can lean on other women for support and for information that can help you to explore your options. If you are open to the idea of receiving support, you are sure to find a community waiting to embrace you.

Next, we will look at some of the specific challenges of IVF and how you can help answer the question, "Am I *Really* Meant to Experience This?"

# CHAPTER THREE

# Am I *Really* Meant To Experience This?

Surely, at some point in your IVF journey, you have asked yourself this difficult question. How is it fair that you've been chosen for this sort of heartache, stress and pain when having children seems to be so easy for everyone else? Chances are, you never imagined that you would be here, doing this.

Before we move on to some of the important tools and strategies to help you get through IVF, I want to first acknowledge what you are going through. Together, the many challenges of infertility make it a struggle like no other.

## Time and Milestones

Part of what makes IVF such a difficult experience is the journey that precedes it. By the time a couple reaches their first IVF cycle, they have been through a wide range of tests, and usually some form of treatment. Along the way, there is usually a good deal of medical speculation about what should work and what may or may not be 'wrong'.

It can be a plodding, indirect advancement. No matter what your age, this long process is very likely to leave you feeling that time is slipping away. As you wait to see doctors, wait for tests and wait for results through each stage of an IVF cycle, you may be acutely aware of time passing.

While you wait, you still have birthdays, celebrate holidays and learn of the pregnancies of others. In other words, you're forced to interact with your world outside of IVF, to acknowledge milestones in your own life and to function as though you are 'fine', even though you may feel distinctly otherwise.

If, like many women, you are older when you reach IVF, you may be even more sensitive to time. Each month can feel like a precious sense of loss. I met Gina through a friend; at age 39, she was feeling less and less control in her life.

> My age is always with me. I know there is nothing that I can do about it, but I feel so trapped. I wish I'd met my husband earlier. I wish we'd started trying right away. I wish we'd arrived at IVF sooner...but, of course, none of that really helps.
>
> —GINA, 39

If you consider yourself to have an advanced maternal age, you are likely to feel a steady sense of pressure. You still deserve to have plenty of hope, however. You have reached the maximum in medical care for fertility issues, and should feel encouraged by the prospects of IVF.

## Emotion and Energy

Perhaps the most pervasive challenge on the road to and through an IVF cycle is the emotional toll that it can take. Although you're not likely to be wrought with emotion all of the time, the months and years of having your hopes rise and fall, of wondering *when* and even *if* it's going to happen for you, can leave you feeling worn.

I met Julie and her husband David in a hospital room, where Julie and I were receiving treatment for our fertility-related immune issues. After trying several medicated Intrauterine Insemination (IUI) cycles, they had recently moved on to IVF. Julie found that her sense of hope was in jeopardy.

> I don't even know if it makes sense to get my hopes up anymore. I'm a bit relieved that we're moving on to IVF, but I don't know if I dare get my hopes up—I'm afraid things might come crashing down.
>
> —Julie, 33

Once an IVF cycle starts, many women find their natural emotions are compounded by the unpredictable effect of fertility drugs. Many times, hope and optimism are coupled with a real fear that they may wind up disappointed yet again.

Often, women fear that if IVF doesn't work the first time, that they will have run out of options. These extremes are entirely common, stressful and exhausting.

## Keeping It Together

One of the most important variables in your experience through IVF is the relationship that you have with your partner.

Because men and women experience and express their feelings so differently, it is important to prioritize your communication with one another. This can be a distinct challenge.

In my own experience, I found that Paul and I needed to find a comfortable balance for the way in which we discussed our fertility efforts. I could have talked about 'what if' and 'let's try this route' all day, every day. Paul was supportive, but always preferred a conversation in which he could identify a solution.

I learned to limit the amount of time that I talked about our fertility issues. When I needed to rant, speculate or even obsess, I often turned to my closest friends or my online support groups.

In time, I learned that in order to communicate effectively with Paul, I had to openly tell him what I needed from him. I needed him to support me in the time and effort that I spent looking for answers. I needed him to understand that I was experiencing things differently than he was. Sometimes, I needed him to just listen without offering solutions.

In turn, I needed to understand that he was experiencing his own, difficult emotions. Although Paul wasn't talking openly about his hopes, fears and frustrations, they were just as much a part of his life as my emotions were a part of mine.

You and your husband will build your own pattern of communication and support. It is an effort, however, and can bring new, difficult dynamics to your marriage. If it feels like your relationship is under steady stress or that you have truly disconnected with one another, consider seeking the support of a professional counselor.

## Managing Logistics

For many women, the logistics of an IVF cycle can be a source of great stress. There are plenty of times during a cycle when it is simply not practical to slip off somewhere for an injection, or to cart along an ice pack to keep your drugs cool. Between having to coordinate injections, clinic appointments, your work schedule and social life, it is easy to feel that IVF has simply taken over.

Depending on the nature of your work, it can also be tricky to manage time off that is sporadic and inconvenient. In my research, teachers, employees of small companies and those whose jobs are unpredictably busy have the most difficulty arranging for time off of work. This is particularly true if their employer is unaware of their medical situation.

This leads to another logistical issue. Given the awkward time requirements of IVF, most women have to make a difficult decision between telling their employer the truth or coming up with a creative string of lies. No matter what kind of relationship you have with your boss or manager, these options can feel uncomfortable and even risky.

Stacey faced the dilemma of how much to tell her employer. As a lawyer, she was expected to put in long hours. As a new employee, she was hesitant to share the fact that she was going through IVF.

> I didn't want to wait to try IVF just because the timing wasn't perfect. On the other hand, trying to keep it hidden from my boss is a huge stress. I'm still debating how much to tell her.
>
> —STACEY, 37

The decision to share your news can bring a great sense of relief. Once your boss knows that you are going through IVF, you can then explain why you may be late to work many mornings, or why you will need time off on short notice for tests or procedures. Of course, every woman who decides to take this route runs the risk that her news will not be supported, perhaps the most difficult situation of all.

Interestingly, I've met several women who found that their jobs seemed to get busier and more stressful, just as they were starting an IVF cycle. I have experienced this myself, and I must admit that the timing of project issues, the resurfacing of thorny colleagues or uncomfortable new assignments can seem almost uncanny.

The social logistics of an IVF cycle can be just as demanding as those faced at work. In truth, your effort to have a baby is nobody's business but your own. You and your partner deserve complete privacy if you choose to keep it to yourselves. Unfortunately, the decision isn't always that simple.

There will very likely be times when you want or need to tell certain people about your cycle. Some women find themselves sharing their news in hopes to get a friend or family member 'off their back' about when they plan to have children. Others decide that they would rather share their news than make excuses to a nosey co-worker about their new work schedule.

> I didn't want to go out for dinner with friends when I would have to cart along my drugs. I wasn't about to make weekend plans when I wasn't sure about the timing of my retrieval. I felt so captive and resentful.
>
> —ANITA, 28

For some women, the logistics of a cycle are made even more complex by distance. Although many women are lucky enough to have their choice of clinics locally, others need to travel to receive treatment. I've even met dedicated couples that have traveled thousands of miles to go through an IVF cycle at a specific clinic. Clearly, this is no small commitment.

## Finding Direction

For some patients of IVF, one of the most frustrating aspects of treatment is simply deciding which direction to take. Because there are wide variations in standards and procedures within the fertility industry, many women are left wondering which way to turn.

Unlike some other medical conditions, where you can expect treatment to be very similar from one doctor to the next, IVF patients often hear very different views on their condition from one clinic to the next.

If you had a poor response to the drugs and a failed cycle, for example, one doctor may push you to consider donor eggs, while another would first want to try a cycle with a different drug protocol. Chances are, if you consulted five specialists about your situation, you would have three or four views on how best to proceed.

Part of the reason for these differing opinions is that the science of fertility is still in its early stages. Although there are promising advances made every year, the industry is also without a set of widely accepted standards.

Most clinics follow their own set of guidelines. Many doctors and clinics conduct their own studies, or are part of research groups that practice specific tests or protocols.

These differences can be enormously frustrating when you want to move ahead and invest yourself emotionally in a single direction. I met Shelley online, after she had done two IVF cycles. When she learned that her second cycle had failed, she wanted to plan out next steps right away.

> I don't know what to do. I know that my clinic
> will push me to consider donor eggs, but I'm just
> not sure that I'm ready for it. I went ahead with
> consultations with two new clinics and all three
> believe that they know just what to do. It's
> expensive to start guessing who is right.
> —SHELLEY, 35

Differing opinions on your situation are not exclusive to fertility clinics. If you choose to look into them, there are plenty of alternative therapies that claim to have reproductive benefits.

Traditional Chinese Medicine (TCM), naturopathy, reiki, crystal healing and hypnotherapy are just a few of the practices that focus on your total well-being and may suggest that they can help you to conceive. Across these therapies, you are likely to find a wide range of suggested diets, treatments, vitamins and lifestyle adjustments.

In my own travels, I consulted with doctors of TCM and naturopaths who specialized in fertility. Their approaches were quite different, yet both were as convinced as my RE that their methods would provide me with my very best chance of becoming pregnant. While their words were encouraging, I could also feel my frustration growing—I longed for a single direction that I could believe in and follow.

Whether you decide to stick with traditional medicine or to investigate alternative therapies, you will encounter differing opinions as you broaden your scope of consultations. It becomes clear very quickly that you are truly in charge of your own direction. This can be empowering, but it can also leave you feeling helpless.

Finding your own best direction may not be a black and white exercise. You may end up combining therapies or using parts of several. You will do well to read as much as you can, consult with your RE on your ideas and let your instinct guide you.

## Difficult Waiting

Any woman who has made it to an IVF cycle knows that there is plenty of waiting involved just to get to your 'day zero', when your follicles will begin to mature. Given that you felt 'ready' to become pregnant long before your first meeting with a doctor, the time leading up to day zero can seem drawn out and tedious.

What is arguably more difficult, however, is the waiting that lies within an IVF cycle itself. Although these periods are short, they can be enormously difficult. Over and over, I have heard women agree that the most challenging parts of an IVF cycle are those brief periods when they are waiting to receive news from their clinic.

I spoke to Kathleen just before her egg retrieval. Already weary from waiting and worrying, she had plenty of difficult waiting ahead.

> I feel so powerless. I hang on every word that the nurse utters. Even though things have gone well so far, the phone calls make me a nervous wreck. I always wish that I had asked better questions. The waiting is torturous.
>
> —KATHLEEN, 32

There are three primary periods of waiting in a fresh IVF cycle. The first begins once you start taking the stimulation drugs to help your eggs to mature. This can be the first moment of truth. After all this time and money spent, is your body reacting as it is supposed to? Depending on the procedures of your clinic, the news of your response to the drugs may be immediate or you may have to wait several hours.

The second period of waiting comes between your egg retrieval and the embryo or blastocyst transfer. Although you will typically know how many eggs were retrieved on the day of the retrieval, the news about fertilization and the progress of your embryos will unfold slowly over the next few days.

As you wait anxiously for each call from the clinic, you may suddenly feel as though everything is beyond your control. At least you had some sense of input when you were giving your-self the injections to help your eggs mature. Now, all you can do is wait and hope. It may feel as though the little ones are 'out there', under the control of others.

The third waiting period is perhaps the most difficult of all. Known as the 'two-week wait', it is the time between your embryo or blastocyst transfer and the clinic's pregnancy test. This can be a torturous, lonely time. For many women, it is the most challenging period of the IVF experience.

During my first cycle, I found the two-week wait to be even more difficult than I had predicted. After a few days, I felt isolated by the sudden lack of interaction with the clinic. I realized that I felt vulnerable and ill-equipped to just be 'on my own' for two challenging weeks.

While you are waiting and hoping, you are also worrying and wondering. Whether you are pregnant or not, your body is going through hormonal changes and adjustments. There are all sorts of twinges, pulls, cramps and symptoms that could be con-strued either way. It is an emotionally charged wait with very lit-tle reprieve.

I met Justine during my second IVF cycle, as she was in the middle of her first. It was clear that she was working hard to make time pass. She was trying to keep busy through her two-week wait, but still found the waiting very difficult.

> I think I'm going crazy. I don't even know if it's the hormones or just the anxiety, but I'm losing it. I feel like I'm stuck in limbo until the (pregnancy) test. If I could only know if it's 'yes' or 'no', I could move on.
>
> —JUSTINE, 36

The waiting that naturally exists within IVF can seem long and difficult. After all that you've committed to have a cycle work, you have a tremendous amount riding on the results. Whether you choose to keep yourself busy during this time or prefer to simply lay low, this component of IVF can test your patience and your nerves.

## Financial Commitment

A list of what makes IVF difficult would not be complete without mention of its financial strain. For most couples, the costs are a significant challenge. IVF can force couples to make emotional decisions around money that can be unexpected and stressful.

Short term, a couple often needs to sacrifice other objectives or even borrow money to pay for a cycle. More than forcing them to examine their priorities, this strain can bring to light some fundamental differences in the way that a couple views and handles money. For some, these differences can lead to a steady source of tension.

I met several women who saw the cost of IVF in terms of the trade-offs that they were making. They described practical sacrifices that would directly affect their lives.

This is eight or nine mortgage payments for us.
—KIM, 31

We'll be doing this instead of any renovations or major repairs on the house this year.
—CARRIE, 40

We really need to replace our car—this is about the cost of a good used car. It's hard.
—JENNIFER, 34

Although none of the women thought that these trade-offs weren't worth making, their honesty shows just how significant the costs can be.

In the longer term, the financial constraints are challenging because they limit the number of times that a couple can realistically attempt to have children that are biologically their own. I've met many women who knew from the outset that they would only be able to afford one cycle. These limitations are realistic and naturally add an extra degree of pressure to a given cycle.

Margaret was in just this situation. She and her husband Dave had endured a long, expensive journey to reach IVF. Having been through seven failed IUI cycles, they had drained their insurance funding and their savings. They agreed that they would try IVF once before considering adoption.

We knew that this was it. I tried to remain as positive as possible, but it was hard not to feel the pressure of a single cycle. I feel so lucky that we beat the odds and had success with our only IVF attempt.
—MARGARET, 37

When it comes to IVF, most couples need to find some sort of balance between time and financial preparation. Some prefer to take the time to set the funds aside, while others want to get on with a cycle and will worry about paying for it later. No matter how you handle money, it is sure to be a factor in how you approach IVF, both practically and emotionally.

## One Thing On Top of Another

Perhaps most noticeable over time, is that the challenges of IVF seem to compound. One hurdle at a time might be easier to navigate, but the way that IVF unfolds, they seem to land in your life all at once.

The drugs used to manipulate your hormones can leave you feeling exhausted and emotional. As your body is reacting to the physical changes, your mind is likely busy, as well.

You may flip back and forth, concentrating on every little twinge you feel in your body, then wondering how you will get away from work over the next few mornings, then struggling with the enormity of the cost if the cycle doesn't work. This new pattern of feelings can take a significant toll.

When I met Julie, she had just finished her first IVF cycle. She was worn out from an accumulation of stress.

> I knew that it would be busy, but I couldn't get over the way that IVF spread through my life. The rush of emotions with each phone call from the clinic, keeping my stories straight at work—I just didn't know it would all be that tiring.
>
> —JULIE, 33

Other women are less aware of the stress they are experiencing. Some stumble through a cycle without a true appreciation for the physical and emotional trials they are under. Patricia did just this. She went through her first IVF cycle with what appeared to be relative ease.

> The shots weren't that bad...worth it, I thought.
> I was able to take things pretty much in stride
> as I worked things around my shots. I definitely
> had fear that it wouldn't work, but I tried to
> think positively as much as possible. When my
> (pregnancy) test was negative, I quickly unraveled.
> —PATRICIA, 29

Patricia's reaction is entirely common. The elation of finally reaching IVF had brought her closer to her goal than ever before. The logistics and hormones of the cycle didn't seem like trouble if it meant that she would soon be pregnant. When she received the negative outcome, however, she began to realize how much stress her mind and body had been under.

So often, the toll of IVF is not just one thing at a time. It is everything, all at once. Many women put on a brave face for themselves, for their partners and even for their friends and family. Meanwhile, it can seem like a long journey with no safe place to rest.

## Coming to Terms With It All

With the many trials of IVF in mind, it is easy to see why so many of us ask, "Am I really meant to experience this?" Getting to and through an IVF cycle is a true test of strength.

You should be proud of yourself for pursuing advanced treatment. Clearly, you value your goal of having a baby so highly that you're willing to sacrifice and persevere, even when it is difficult to do so.

Personally, I found the most comforting answer to this question to be, "Yes, I am meant to experience this." I didn't see why it was happening, and there were certainly days when I felt tested beyond my ability to cope, but it did help to think that for some reason this experience was meant to be part of my life.

No matter how you answer this question in your own mind, it will help to acknowledge that a fertility struggle brings a wide range of challenges to your life. It is likely to change the way you see the world around you and how you interact socially. Perhaps your greatest challenge is to ensure that it doesn't have a negative impact on the way you see yourself.

Throughout the remaining chapters, we will take a closer look at some of the ways you can mitigate the challenges of IVF by learning to put yourself first. We will start with a brief look at a concept that is an important part of nurturing yourself through IVF: making the most of your personal energy.

# CHAPTER FOUR

# Understanding Your Energy

WHEN IT COMES TO IMPROVING your experience through IVF, it is helpful to start with an understanding of your personal energy. Your energy is not simply a description of how much 'get up and go' you have, nor is it a reflection of your initiative or stamina.

It is directly connected to something much more personal: your thoughts and feelings, and how they are reflected in your physical conditions. The things you do and say, the beliefs you hold and the way in which your internal dialogue unfolds are all important contributors to your energy.

Although it requires an effort to understand how your energy plays itself out in your life, it is important work for one simple reason: the better you are able to make your experience through IVF, the more likely you are to have success.

While this may sound simplistic for such a complex subject, it is a powerful truth. It is rooted in the direct connection between your mind and body, and it is at the heart of nurturing yourself through IVF.

## Your Mind-Body Connection

The mind-body connection is well documented and widely recognized by the medical community. Best described as the ability of your thoughts to influence your biology, the mind-body connection is cited again and again as people overcome illness, live past their life expectations or surpass other medical challenges.

The mind-body connection is based on the notion that your thoughts, feelings and emotions directly affect the ability of your body to operate at its peak efficiency.

**What You Can Do!**
To learn more about how the mind-body connection relates to fertility, read Dr. Alice Domar's book, *Conquering Infertility*. See "Appendix One: A Few Great Resources."

It has been proven that people who make an effort to think positively, those who use hypnotherapy, meditation or other means to intentionally guide their thoughts, are able to directly impact their bodies on a cellular level.

For women going through IVF, this is a powerful concept. Because so many fertility issues are based on imbalances of one or more of our internal systems, the idea that we can affect biological changes is both promising and empowering. Even women facing 'unexplained infertility' or 'male factor' alone can help to make their bodies more receptive to pregnancy through mind-body techniques.

Although it may sound simple to start thinking positively, it can be a difficult change to make. Using your thoughts to

positively influence your biology requires a steady commitment, a regular process of 'letting go' and a willingness to
truly believe that changes are coming.

Karen had turned to mind-body techniques to help her
through her third IVF cycle. After feeling that the first two
cycles had drained her energy and weakened her spirit, she
enrolled in a 12-week program designed to reduce stress and
enhance fertility.

> I thought I would give it a shot. It sounded
> like an easy thing to do and I needed to try
> something to make a difference. After just a
> couple of sessions, I realized that letting go of
> the stress I'd been carrying around would take
> work. It does get easier over time, but it takes
> commitment.
>
> —KAREN, 36

In combination with her IVF treatment and mind-body techniques, Karen was able to achieve a successful pregnancy. She
credits fate, luck, God, good doctors and a healthy mind-body
balance for her eventual success.[1]

## A Better Balance

When you start to learn more about the mind-body connection, you will see how its benefits can carry a positive momen-
tum. The more you are able to 'let go', the more stress you will
release, the better you will feel and the better balance you will
achieve.

---

[1] Karen attended the Mind-Body Fertility Program in Toronto, Canada:
www.conceivethepossibility.com.

With respect to IVF, a healthy balance between mind and body can provide an important advantage. Consider the following relationship:

> improved experience =
> improved personal energy (feelings, emotions) =
> improved body conditions =
> improved odds of success

Clearly, this logic is an expansion of the mind-body connection and illustrates how something as simple as your thoughts can help to improve your odds for success. When you are able to monitor your internal dialogue, treat yourself gently and proceed with a calm, positive outlook, you will be much better positioned for success.

If you are interested in learning more about the mind-body connection, especially as it relates to fertility, there are plenty of resources available online. Start by entering "mind-body infertility" into a search engine, or see "Appendix One: A Few Great Resources" for further ideas.

## Finding Stability

Even if you don't feel quite prepared to do further research, please trust that your personal energy does matter as you go through IVF. Your energy and experience are closely connected. They are largely controlled by you and your thoughts.

Where you are willing to make positive changes in how you speak to yourself and how you allow yourself to truly unwind, you will be bettering your health and naturally improving your odds for success. With an appreciation for *your* role in your experience through IVF, you will better be able to make these positive changes.

Next, we will look at how the inherent highs and lows of an IVF cycle can affect our personal energy. We will see just how we can begin to replace negative or doubtful thoughts with ones that provide more stability and positive energy. Being aware of, and deliberate with, our feelings is a great place to start.

# CHAPTER FIVE

# Embracing Your
# Natural Advantage

IF YOU WERE TOLD THAT YOU HAVE a natural advantage in becoming pregnant, you might not believe it. An advantage might seem like a bit of a stretch when you've had to confront more challenges than most people would ever need to consider.

Although it is very likely buried beneath layers of doubt, disappointment and anxiety, rest assured that you do indeed have a natural advantage that you can cultivate and strengthen.

Simply put, your advantage is based on your heart's desire. You've known for some time just how much you want to conceive and carry a baby to term. That part is easy. It is a clear goal; it is loving and incredibly powerful. You can take heart knowing that your goal provides a built-in head start; it is your natural advantage.

**If knowing my goal is such an advantage, why hasn't it helped so far?**

This is a fair question—one that requires us to take a closer look at how a natural advantage can exist in our lives. Quite simply, it does not exist on its own. It is a thought, deep within us, surrounded by plenty of other thoughts, feelings and emotions.

As you might imagine, it is supported and strengthened by feelings such as hope, love, happiness and optimism. It is suppressed by feelings such as fear, doubt and sadness.

Your natural advantage works best when your feelings are level, calm and consistent. It is challenged by feelings that are volatile or inconsistent. If you have been stumbling along from one feeling to another, you may have been inadvertently making your own experience more difficult than it needs to be. The very good news is that your natural advantage is easily influenced and can be improved with even the smallest effort.

## Accidental Energy

Naturally, your path to and through IVF will be marked with a wide range of strong emotions. As you move back and forth between feelings of hope and fear, between joy and overwhelming doubt, there are consequences for your mind and body— your natural advantage takes a bit of a beating.

Think of what happens when you pass a mother with her newborn on the street. If you're like many women, your initial reaction is warm and appreciative. Almost immediately, however, these feelings can flash to envy or sadness.

Why her? Does she even appreciate what she has? Will it ever happen for me?

Your thoughts may run a wide range between happiness, hope and utter misery. All the while, your body is listening and reacting.

34

The wide range of feelings, the rapid change between one extreme and another—these are normal experiences, caused by something that I call accidental energy.

Accidental energy is simply experience without deliberate consciousness. Because it has little resistance to circumstances or mood swings, changes between feelings can be sudden and unwelcome. When an emotional challenge causes us to feel up at times and down at others, accidental energy usually prevails.

One of the reasons that accidental energy is so common through an IVF cycle is that you are often at the mercy of a turbulent internal dialogue. Without being conscious of the pattern, most women going through IVF simply follow whichever thoughts or emotions present themselves next. Very often, this results in an uncomfortable pattern of energy.

Tara had just this situation. I met Tara and Jeff when they had been trying to conceive for two and a half years. They were just approaching their first IVF cycle, having suffered the disappointment of three failed IUI cycles the year before.

Both were feeling cautiously optimistic, but Tara confessed to wide swings between her feelings; she found it challenging to remain positive:

> At last, after all this waiting...this is it, we're going to have a baby!

> What if it doesn't work? What on earth will I do?

> Would it help if I took certain vitamins or herbs?

> What if we're missing a test that we should have had before spending the money on IVF?

This sort of dialogue can take you for a bumpy ride. Without an awareness of how your thoughts and feelings impact you, you can easily stumble into this unhealthy up and down pattern.

Accidental energy can be hazardous through an IVF cycle because it leaves you vulnerable to your environment. When you are feeling tired, angry or low, you are particularly at risk.

It may seem, for example, that you are suddenly unable to escape your pregnant neighbor who loves to fantasize about your children playing together. Perhaps you hear of a rash of new pregnancies at work or your least favorite colleague drops by to tell you that she is unexpectedly pregnant *again*. It can be easy for a single conversation, moment or insensitive comment to throw you off for a while.

Of course, there only seem to be more of these moments when you are so tuned-in to the subjects of pregnancy, babies and children. The toll they can take is real, however, and they can test your patience, hope and self-esteem.

Without a more deliberate approach, your environment will play a significant role in how you experience IVF. Rather than hoping for 'good' days through a cycle, rather than hoping that your circumstances are not upsetting or difficult, it is important to learn specific skills to level out your emotions, no matter what you encounter.

## Learning to Observe

With an appreciation for the importance of your feelings and emotions, you can begin to observe how they exist in your life. Observing is a loving, non-judgmental role in which you consciously witness the feelings that you have around anything-IVF. It is simply listening-in on your inner-dialogue.

This means monitoring how you feel while driving into the parking lot at your clinic, while preparing your nightly injection, while talking 'sleep and drool' with your co-workers who have young children—anything. Take note when the feelings arrive, how intense they are, and whether or not they are coupled with other feelings.

Once you have been able to observe for a while, start to notice how negative feelings can evolve. Keep in mind that negative feelings have a sneaky way about them. They are often disguised as neutral feelings, and can creep into your inner-dialogue with little notice.

Consider, for example, the number of times that you use phrases such as "I hope this works..." or "This is it—we're doing everything that we can." Although seemingly positive, these thoughts can be laden with doubt and negative energy.

As you monitor your inner-dialogue, you will likely notice that fear and doubt, two of the most common emotions through an IVF journey, have an unpleasant feel to them. They are among the most negative feelings that you can experience, and they can wreak havoc on your personal energy.

Rest assured, I am not suggesting that you do away with negative feelings by sugar-coating them with happy, giddy feelings. Rather, I want to suggest that once you have an awareness of how negative feelings exist in your life, you will be in a better position to lessen their impact.

With even the smallest effort, you can begin to replace your negative thoughts, the down-side of your accidental energy, with more level, calm energy.

## Becoming Deliberate

If level, positive energy is our goal, we need to first learn how to become more deliberate with our experience, our thoughts, feelings and emotions. As we will see throughout the remaining chapters, there are many ways to do so.

In Chapter Six, "Being Kind to Yourself," we will see a few ways to give yourself a well-deserved break through IVF.

In Chapter Seven, "Finding Your Life Raft," we will see how a sense of physical calm and a process of mentally letting go through relaxation and other techniques can help you to gain a greater sense of control over your mind and body.

In Chapter Eight, "Editing the World Around You," we will see specific ways to become more deliberate with your environment. In a society that generally assumes that it is easy for a woman to become pregnant, it is important to have a set of coping skills to keep your positive energy in tact.

Finally, in Chapter Nine, "Creating Your New To-Do List," we will look at things that you can do to proactively improve your peace of mind and your odds of success.

By taking action in these ways, you are sure to gain a sense of empowerment. As you are more aware of your thoughts and feelings and are willing to deliberately make them more steady, calm and positive, your personal energy will surely improve. Over time, you will steadily lessen the effect of accidental energy in your life.

## But, But, But

I want to address a concern that may be lingering in your mind. If you are like many women going through fertility treatment, you may feel skeptical that changing your energy will be enough to overcome your particular challenges. This may be especially true if you have been through IVF more than once, or if your fertility issues include known physical or biological barriers.

I understand completely. I was also very doubtful when I first started reading about the importance of feelings and energy. I believed that changing my feelings could probably make a difference in some areas of life, but not in my fertility situation.

If you do feel skeptical that changing your personal energy will be enough to overcome your fertility challenges, consider this: it is relatively simple to do, it is healthy for your mind and body, and it is more or less free.

Perhaps most important, it can help you to weather the ups and downs of IVF, giving you the energy and clarity to ask the right questions and pursue new ideas. With peace of mind and with your emotions level, you will better be able to answer questions such as:

~ *Are we ready to try an IVF cycle?*

~ *Should we try to convince our doctor to try a new protocol, or is it time for us to consider changing clinics?*

~ *Are we willing to try another IVF cycle, or is it time for us to move on to other paths to parenthood?*

These are serious questions; their impact is both far-reaching and highly personal. You will do well to tackle these kinds of decisions with a sense of calm and confidence.

Before discounting the ability of your personal energy to help in *your* situation, I urge you to read on with an open mind. Changing your energy *can* have an unexplainable, positive result in your IVF experience. If this seems significant and hopeful, it should.

## Your Natural Advantage Grows

The goal in this chapter has been two-fold: to introduce you to the idea of your natural advantage (your clear, powerful goal of having a baby) and to illustrate how it is subject to the ups and downs of your emotions (your accidental energy).

As we've seen, your natural advantage is extremely powerful, but slightly delicate. It needs to be consciously supported, both within your daily routine and when you are caught off-guard by difficult situations. By tuning in to your inner-dialogue and putting a halt to negative thought patterns, you will gradually gain a sense of control over your accidental energy.

With commitment, an open mind and some patience with yourself, you can learn to increase the control that you feel over your emotions and your personal energy. And so your natural advantage, your built-in head start, grows.

Next, we will look at a few of the most important ways that you can treat yourself well during this time. You deserve to catch a break now and then; sometimes, you need to be the one to give it to yourself.

# CHAPTER SIX

# Being Kind to Yourself

An important part of nurturing yourself through IVF is learning how to treat yourself with kindness. Kindness means gentle, patient and forgiving treatment. It means letting yourself off the hook as often as possible, and realizing that you don't have to be perfect through this difficult journey.

## Letting it All Out

Although this book encourages positive and hopeful thinking, I want to also acknowledge that you will have days when you feel anything but positive. Every woman who has gone through an IVF cycle can attest that there are good days, mediocre days and some very bad days. It is entirely normal to have days when all sense of hope seems to escape you.

Beyond the obvious times that can trigger setbacks (family parties, birthdays and holidays), there can be days that feel like a challenge for no reason at all. You're tired of waiting, you're tired of trying to be positive, you're simply tired of it all.

Part of being kind to yourself includes having a willingness to 'let it all out' on occasion. Sometimes you need to simply acknowledge that this whole thing stinks.

It's rotten that you have to go through IVF. It stinks that you have to worry about whether or not it will work. Be sad, scream and have an all-day cry if you need to—it is a healing, natural exercise to let these feelings go.

Even if you are doing your best to remain positive through IVF, it is natural to feel like you have fallen down at times. Be easy on yourself. Take some time to acknowledge just how hard all of this is. Allow yourself some time to regroup and to feel good about your plans.

Just a word of caution: if you find that you are having more bad days than good, or if it feels like 'too much' most of the time, it may be time to seek some guidance. I am not a counselor, but I know that there are real benefits to discussing your feelings with a professional.

Most fertility clinics either have professional counselors on staff or can help you to find these services locally. If you are feeling overwhelmed or have persistent feelings of anxiety, irritation or anger, this may be just the outlet that you need.

## Forgive, Forgive, Forgive

Another part of being kind to yourself involves creating a sense of forgiveness for both yourself and others. Given the frustrating nature of a fertility struggle, it is easy to have feelings of resentment, guilt or anger spill over into almost all areas of your life. The more you are able to recognize how these feelings affect you, the easier it will be to let them go through forgiveness.

If you are like many women going through IVF, forgiveness may need to start with yourself. Through my research, I found that women commonly wondered if they had done something in the past to damage their fertility. Some also wondered if they somehow deserved the challenges they were facing.

Quite simply, this is not your fault. It is highly unlikely that anything that either you or your partner have done would result in a fertility struggle. You do not deserve this; it's just where you have landed.

Perhaps more challenging than forgiving ourselves is the effort required to forgive others. When you're in the middle of fertility struggle, issues at home and at work can seem bigger and more aggravating than they might otherwise.

It may suddenly seem that family, friends and co-workers feel compelled to make insensitive, thoughtless comments about pregnancy, babies or children. Whether or not your community knows about your efforts to become pregnant, they may say things that make you feel terrible.

I met Elaine on my train ride to work. Shortly after we became acquainted with one another, we realized that we faced similar fertility struggles. Over time, it became apparent that Elaine's journey was made increasingly painful by the comments of her family.

> My in-laws know that we are going through
> IVF—it's no secret. Last weekend, my
> mother-in-law pointed out a corner of the
> living room where we could put a playpen,
> and went on to tell me how her friends are
> about to become first-time grandmothers.
> I wanted to strangle her.
> —ELAINE, 35

Thankfully, Elaine has a terrific sense of humor and could use it as a coping tool. If you find that your own humor wears thin, you may be left with nothing but frustration or anger. In this case, forgiveness can work wonders. If you are able to let offending people off the hook to some degree, you will greatly lessen the impact of their comments.

Perhaps the perpetrators in your life are oblivious to what you are going through. If they do know, maybe they just don't know what to say. Let's face it, there is very little that anyone could say that would be of comfort, and maybe they are just stumbling along trying to say anything at all.

If it will help you to forgive others, consider helping them to understand just what you are going through. Send them web sites, point them to articles or books. Do whatever you can to help them simply know better.

In her light-hearted, pragmatic personal web site called So Close, Tertia writes web logs about all things related to infertility and life in general. Having been through IVF herself, she recommends that we educate people around us as a way of helping ourselves.

> **If we can get just one person to stop saying 'just relax' we will have helped the sisterhood.**[2]

Forgiveness is a very calming, healthy act. While it is not always easy or realistic, the more you are able to let go of negative feelings, the better you will feel.

## Surround Yourself With Greatness

One very empowering way to be kind to yourself through IVF is to build a top-notch support team. Be warned, this requires a conscious effort to make changes in the list of people

---

[2] http://tertia.typepad.com/so_close (*So Close: Surviving Infertility*)

with whom you associate. It means having a willingness to part with negative or toxic relationships and to gravitate toward those that are positive and healthy.

Consider the people in your life who know about your efforts to have children. If you are like most of us, you have a few positive, empathic people nearby who truly care about you. You may also have a handful of relationships that feel just the opposite—those with people who are negative, selfish or unwilling to try and understand what you are going through.

Naturally, you will be at a great advantage if you can gravitate towards the people who support you most. Where possible, do away with negative or toxic relationships. Although this isn't always easy, especially if the difficult relationship is with a family member, it is very rewarding. If it is too complicated or would take too long to actually sever the relationship, consider simply avoiding these people while you are going through IVF.

Perhaps most tricky to manage, are the relationships that fall somewhere between positive and negative. Can you think of people who leave you feeling drained or down after you interact with them? Perhaps they have a tendency to make you feel guilty, or seem to somehow feed off of your energy.

These relationships can be just as damaging as those that are overtly negative. Because it is so important to put yourself first through IVF, consider parting ways with these people for a while, too.

Once you make a conscious effort to spend your time with supportive friends and family members, you will very likely feel a sense of relief. This is a sure sign that you've made the right decisions about who to 'keep', and who to 'let go'.

## Give Yourself a Break

Perhaps one of the most obvious ways to be kind to yourself is one that is difficult for most of us to do. It is simply to take a break.

Although it can be hard to take a break between cycles when you are concerned about the passage of time, it is an important reprieve. It is an opportunity for you to shake off some pressure, release yourself from the steady flow of strong emotions and get back to yourself for a while.

I've met over a dozen women who, when forced to take a break for financial, logistical or other reasons were relieved for the change. Keira, one of these women, was openly thrilled.

> I'm so happy for a little time with my husband that isn't all about fertility. I'll get back into it all when I need to, but for now, bring on the wine. I need a break.
>
> —KEIRA, 36

When I was forced to take a break between cycles, I decided to run in a 10K race. It was against my RE's better judgment to exercise heavily while trying to become pregnant, but I didn't care. I needed to do something that was just for me. The race was on a beautiful spring day—I felt full of life and fabulous as I ran as fast as I could.

If you find yourself with an option to take a break, consider it as an opportunity to have time for yourself. Even one month can give you the chance to regroup, revitalize and to approach your next cycle with a more positive outlook.

## Kindness Begets Kindness

There are many ways to be kind to yourself as you go through IVF. Your best strategies for doing so will be based on your likes, interests and circumstances. You will likely need to be proactive, creating opportunities for self-kindness as you go.

Your efforts will be fruitful, however. As you experiment with ways to be kind to yourself, you are sure to come across new ideas. Embrace each opportunity as it arrives—you deserve to feel relieved and happy as much as possible.

Next, we will look at some useful ways to further improve your odds of IVF success. Anything you can do to bring stillness or peace of mind to your life at this time will improve your experience and your health. Fortunately, there are plenty of ways to help you let go and bring stillness to your active mind.

# CHAPTER SEVEN
# Finding Your Life Raft

CONSIDERING THE TRIALS OF IVF, a life raft might sound like a good idea. Anything that will help you to feel a greater sense of control is worth pursuing. An IVF life raft should provide you with both a physical and a mental escape. It should allow you to feel that you are whole and happy. In short, it should help you to feel like the woman you were before having a baby even crossed your mind.

My own realization that I needed a life raft came over me suddenly. Tired of waiting for success, I had grown accustomed to the unwelcome feelings of sadness, frustration and a sense of emptiness.

These emotions were never part of my life before we started trying to have children, yet somehow they had become my constant companions. I wanted desperately to be 'free' again—to laugh until it hurt, to truly forget about it all for a while and embrace life rather than feel like everything was always on hold.

Fortunately, I did stumble across a life raft that worked wonders in my IVF journey. It was simple, but incredibly powerful. It
was the ability to proactively and consistently create an inner
sense of calm through some of the relaxation techniques that will
be covered in this chapter.

Over time, I could see that once I gave myself the time and
permission to enjoy a sense of calm, it could provide both short
and long-term benefits. I learned to love the immediate sense of
release that relaxation allowed.

In a short time, I seemed to be able to shake off a tremendous
amount of frustration and unrest that had accumulated during
the day. This alone felt indulgent and rewarding.

Longer term, I knew that I could greatly improve the condition of my mind and body if I was able to unwind in this way.
Fortunately, it was something that I truly enjoyed.

When all around me seemed busy, stressful or unhappy, I had
my personal time, my relaxation to look forward to. It was truly
my life raft.

I am confident that this simple act can help you through your
IVF experience, as well. Once you learn how to achieve an inner
sense of peace, you will be able to call upon it, during even the
most challenging parts of an IVF cycle.

## What is Stillness?

Stillness is not just the absence of sound or activity. It is not a
quiet drive to work in which you run over your 'to-do' list for
the day. It is not a Saturday morning in which you flop your legs
over the side of the couch to read the paper. Nor is it the time at
night when you are quietly drifting off to sleep.

What stillness *is* may surprise you. It is a sense of inner peace,
quiet and joy. More than something you do, it is a natural state of

being when your body and mind are deeply relaxed; it is what happens when you are able to completely let go.

Deep relaxation allows your body and mind to work together to heal and rebuild. This is a promising notion for any woman going through IVF. It not only provides you with a break from the emotional highs and lows, but has also been proven to help your body operate at its peak efficiency.

There are many ways to find stillness, and we will cover several options here. Keep in mind, however, that you will likely discover your own ways to achieve an inner sense of peace, how and when it is right for you.

## Why We Need to Let Go

When we experience stress, even if the perceived amount is very low, our brains automatically trigger a number of actions. Cortisol, adrenaline and other chemicals are released into our bloodstream, our muscles become tense, our hearts beat faster and our breathing becomes shallow and more rapid.

Over time, even low-level stress can take a significant toll. With increased activity, our nervous system is strained and our adrenal and immune systems become fatigued. Without an opportunity to escape the source of stress and rejuvenate, our bodies are at an increased risk for disease.

Fortunately, our bodies have another automatic function, known as the relaxation response. It occurs when we are deeply relaxed, with a calm internal environment. In this state, we have an incredible ability to combat stress. Our bodies are allowed to rejuvenate, heal and unwind.

While it would be nice if we could automatically create this environment at the end of the day, the reality is that we need to work at this a little. We need to proactively let go, in order for our natural healing to begin.

You may be wondering how realistic it is to relax deeply while in the midst of an IVF cycle. In truth, it *is* a challenge to find the motivation to create a calm internal environment when there are so many demands on your time and energy.

So why not just 'get through' a cycle without the added pressure to be calm? The answer is something that you probably already know—the advantages far outweigh the effort involved.

If you are willing to spend some time and remain open to the possibilities, a sense of calm will serve you well through IVF. You may find motivation in the following list of advantages.

An internal sense of calm can allow you to:

### i) maximize your health and your odds

It is widely known that stress can wreak havoc on our physical health. Almost every system in our body is affected by the hormones and reactions caused by stress, including our reproductive systems.

Dr. Alice Domar, Harvard psychologist and infertility specialist addresses the important role that stress can play in her book, *Conquering Infertility*.

> If you're struggling with infertility, stress creates a vicious circle: You get stressed because you can't conceive, which makes you more stressed, and that makes it even harder to conceive. ...This process can spiral on endlessly unless you learn to break the cycle of stress.[3]

---

[3] Dr. Alice Domar, *Conquering Infertility*. (New York: Viking Penguin, 2002), p. 20.

ıg inner stillness does just this—it allows you to inter-
cycle of stress, counteracting its negative health effects
,proving your odds of success.

## ii) indulge in short-term escape / enjoyment

Let's face it, while we all agree that the end result of holding our babies in our arms will be worth the effort, there is not too much about an IVF cycle that could be considered enjoyable. Indulging in short-term escape through a sense of calm is an effective and inexpensive way to pamper yourself during this busy time.

As you go through the process of mentally letting go, you will be able to remove yourself from outside sources of stress, from thoughts related to work, and from the turbulent inner dialogue that is so often part of a struggle to become pregnant. You may be surprised to find just how enjoyable it is to clear your mind completely.

## iii) use perspective to your advantage

Any journey through IVF is filled with emotional decisions and key turning points. Along your own path, you will regularly be required to make choices that will ultimately impact your experience, your happiness and your success.

As we saw earlier, you may be faced with significant questions that have long-term implications. Which clinic should you use? Should you supplement your treatment with alternative therapies? When is it time to move on to a new clinic, consider a new protocol, or look into new options in becoming parents?

You will always be at a great advantage when you are able to make decisions from a calm, confident perspective.

### iv) build on your success

One of the advantages of learning how to create a sense of calm is that it has a cumulative effect on your mind and body. The more you proactively let go, the easier it becomes, and the greater the impact it has on the rest of your life.

Knowing that you can achieve this inner sense of peace as a reliable way to escape stress, you are likely to find that stress has less impact on you overall. This is a distinct advantage for your journey through IVF.

Hopefully this list of benefits provides you with the motivation to learn more. In practice, it takes effort to make stillness a regular part of your busy life. In order to do so, you will need a reliable set of tools and a realistic plan.

## Your Internal Toolkit

There are a number of techniques to help you to elicit your body's relaxation response. Whether you prefer the structure of a relaxation recording or to spend time quietly on your own, you may need to experiment to find the techniques that fit you best.

As you explore different options in relaxation, try not to feel obliged to concentrate on one style or practice. Relaxation should be calming, refreshing and enjoyable. You shouldn't feel that it is a chore, or just one more thing to get through before the end of the day.

Here are just a few of the techniques that you might first explore:

### Breathing Exercises

If you've ever been to a yoga class, you've likely heard that without thought, we normally breathe into the top one-third of our lungs. When you encounter stress, your lung usage is decreased even further.

When you practice deep, slow abdominal breathing, you bring air into the bottom two-thirds of your lungs. This sort of rhythmical breathing requires a conscious effort, but there are distinct health benefits and the results can be felt almost immediately.

First, deep abdominal breathing helps to trigger your body's relaxation response, your most powerful tool in coping with stress. The combination of the slow, rhythmical movement of your diaphragm and belly, along with reduced strain on your nervous system, helps you to truly, deeply relax.

Another important advantage is purely physical. Deep breathing requires up-and-down movements of your diaphragm and creates in-and-out movements in your belly, ribcage and lower back. This movement helps to massage your inner organs, it helps your lymph system to operate more efficiently, and it promotes blood flow throughout your body.

Finally, because deep breathing requires a focused effort, it can become an exercise in mental distraction, as well. It is difficult to focus on much else when you are visualizing the movement of your breath.

Used properly, deep breathing can become an effective tool in helping your mind to unwind, and can serve as an excellent warm up for further relaxation.

## Relaxation Techniques

The term 'relaxation' is broadly used to cover a wide range of exercises that can elicit your body's relaxation response. Although they differ in structure and format, their objectives are generally the same. Two of the most popular methods of relaxation include:

**progressive relaxation**—In this exercise, you slowly scan your body mentally, tensing and then relaxing specific muscle groups.

**guided relaxation**—Through this technique, you imagine yourself being somewhere specific that is pleasant and relaxing; your body relaxes while you are focusing on the details of your imagined surroundings.

These techniques can be practiced on your own, or with the aid of a recording. Personally, I found that I had too much on my mind through IVF to try to focus on either of these tools without the help of an audio guide.

There are plenty of excellent relaxation recordings available; some are designed specifically to help enhance fertility. "Appendix One: A Few Great Resources" lists several helpful audio recordings.

## Yoga

Rooted in ancient practices of physical and mental discipline, yoga effectively promotes internal harmony by allowing your internal energy to flow and heal. Yoga requires slow movement, deep breathing and a concentrated effort that allows your mind to effectively relax. It is a natural way to release tension and stress.

Among yoga's many health benefits are:

~ increased flexibility

~ internal detoxification

~ joints, ligaments and tendons are lubricated

~ internal organs are massaged

~ nervous system is balanced

I started taking yoga after my first RE advised me to do so. He struck me as a conservative sort, so when he told me to do yoga, "not once, not twice, but three times a week," I took notice. If *he* believed in it, I knew there must be something to it.

After a few classes, I had forgotten that it was good for me— I was simply enjoying it. While I was concentrating on physical movements, I found that my mind relaxed naturally and without effort.

Thankfully, yoga has gained tremendous popularity in western cultures. If you are interested in giving it a try, you will likely be able to find a nearby class with relative ease.

## Meditation

Meditation is another ancient practice that brings about deep relaxation. By keeping your body still and your focus on a specific word, object or goal, your mind is able to block out the clutter and activity of daily life. Regular meditation allows you to create an inner silence that is both healing and nurturing.

Although meditation was not my chosen method of relaxation, I met several women for whom it was. Lisa swore that it was her sanctuary through IVF.

> I don't know if I would say that it is what made IVF work for me, but it definitely helped. For a month leading up to my cycle, and through to my first ultrasound, I would meditate for about 20 minutes with a different word every night. I used words like 'bountiful', 'healthy', and 'fertile'. It was just very peaceful—it was an important time for me.
>
> —LISA, 37

Once you begin to explore relaxation techniques and find the ones that work for you, you will have an internal toolkit that you can rely upon with confidence. Over time, it will get easier to truly let go and enjoy a sense of calm.

You will know that you've found the right set of techniques when you look forward to your sessions, and when you miss a sense of calm when you've had to skip one. Like anything, it can take practice before you can truly enjoy relaxation, but please be patient and expect great rewards.

## Getting Back to Yourself

Finding a life raft through IVF can allow you to feel free and even carefree for a period of time. For many women, these feelings can seem like a distant memory. What happens when you do let go, even for a short time, is that your natural sense of self comes rushing back in.

### I used to be so happy—what happened to that woman?

Through my journey and subsequent research, I was surprised to find the number of women who felt like they had lost part of themselves along their fertility journey. They knew that they had been happy in the past, but couldn't imagine feeling that way in the present. They were sure that they wouldn't truly be happy until they had a baby in their arms.

I certainly felt this way myself. In the early part of my journey, I felt like I had forgotten about true happiness altogether. Every event that passed through my life was seen from the perspective of a woman struggling to have a baby.

Over time, I recognized this feeling as a deep, personal longing to 'get back to myself'. I met Leah, one of the women who shared this feeling, while we were waiting to see a specialist.

> **I feel completely different since starting all of this. My husband and I fight over ridiculous things. I know that I'm irritable, but I just can't help it. I can't imagine being as happy as we were when we were first married.**
>
> —LEAH, 38

Getting back to yourself isn't a selfish goal. It doesn't mean that you want to put aside your goal of having a baby. Instead, it means that you want to be able to reclaim who *you* were before you even thought about having children. It means that you want to be able to live in the moment again, to feel true happiness and contentedness with all that you *do* have.

Like Leah, I had a hard time even remembering what my old self was like. If you feel this way yourself, it may be hard to imagine 'getting back' there at all. I found that learning how to create a sense of inner stillness was a great place to start.

## One Advantage on Top of Another

Whether you are waiting for an IVF cycle to begin or are right in the middle of one, learning how to find a sense of calm can provide you with important advantages. It promotes a sense of control. It allows you to become more deliberate with your feelings. It provides a short-term escape from everything on your mind and offers distinct health benefits.

The list of advantages could go on. If you are willing to keep an open mind and dedicate the time for true relaxation to take place, you will be embracing one of the most valuable tools in nurturing yourself through IVF. You will have found an all-important life raft.

Next, we will look at another way to promote an inner sense of peace. Rather than focusing on your internal world, however, we will turn our attention to the world around us. Learning to distance yourself from parts of your environment can be an important skill when you are working hard to become pregnant.

# CHAPTER EIGHT
# Editing The World Around You

As you begin to develop the skills that we have already covered, you will surely feel your emotions begin to level out. Even as your skills improve, however, there will be plenty of events, situations and comments that can catch you off-guard.

Here, we will learn another important skill: how to 'turn off' or 'edit' parts of your environment to help you through these difficult times. Editing the world around you involves making conscious decisions about how to handle social situations, how to react to uncomfortable moments, and above all, how to protect yourself through your entire IVF journey.

If it sounds difficult to simply turn off parts of the world around you, it is. Work and social commitments are part of what make you a functioning member of society. It is not realistic to think that you would experience a difficult fertility journey without external challenges.

With some simple tools and a sense of self-awareness, however, you will be able to increase your confidence, improve your peace of mind and generally improve your experience through IVF. As you grow more skilled at editing the world around you, you will naturally become more deliberate with your energy.

## Identifying Triggers

One of the most useful ways to get through the more challenging parts of IVF is to identify events and situations that trigger negative feelings. Although it is ideal to identify these scenarios ahead of time, there will likely be times that you stumble across these triggers as you go.

The good news is that once you are aware of your personal energy and how it is affected by your feelings, it does gradually get easier to spot trigger situations in advance. You can probably think of a few of these situations already.

Some of the most common include:

~ a friend or family member announcing her pregnancy

~ co-workers or friends engaging in 'baby-talk'—talking at length about their pregnancies or young children

~ being asked by new acquaintances if you have children

~ being around people who you know are wondering, "When the heck are they going to have kids?"

~ just being around friends and family over the holidays

The list really could go on and on. You will certainly have your own personal triggers. These situations can quickly bring on strong feelings such as sadness, resentment or a sense of emptiness. They can also result in feelings that are more subtle, but equally as damaging.

I met Sharon when she was suffering from the sting of a recent miscarriage. Her pregnancy had followed a long fertility journey, and she was understandably devastated by the loss. It was the beginning of the holiday season, and Sharon realized that she faced a long series of trigger events ahead.

> I don't want to be around anyone with kids or babies, not even my family. I just want to crawl into a hole and be alone. I can't pretend to be happy and fine right now.
> —SHARON, 31

Beth was just as aware of a known trigger in her life. I met Beth at work; she regularly told me how just being in the presence of her sister-in-law made her uncomfortable. Her brother's wife was younger and became pregnant as soon as they started trying to have children.

> Every time we see her, she talks about how easy it was for her to become pregnant. Even though she knows what we're going through, she overdoes the baby talk around their son. I always end up leaving their place feeling mad.
> —BETH, 30

If, like Sharon and Beth, you are able to identify your own trigger events, you will be better able to handle them. When you have time to prepare yourself in advance, you can develop specific skills that will help you to react with a sense of calm resolution.

## Choose Your Response

If you do have advance warning of a trigger event, you usually have at least three options in terms of how you react. In order to illustrate, consider the following example:

*You've been invited to Thanksgiving dinner, where you suspect that your younger, newly-married cousin will be announcing her pregnancy to the family. This will be the first grandchild for your aunt and uncle, and you know that they will be ecstatic.*

*Your cousin has been hinting for the last year that the two of you should become pregnant at the same time—it is all but certain that she will bring this up again at the dinner table. You're in the middle of a frustrating waiting period in your own fertility journey and can't imagine how you will handle this dinner.*

The very act of anticipating an uncomfortable social event is likely a familiar exercise. Here are some possible reactions to the news of your invitation:

### i) Let dread rule the day

The most common reaction to this scenario is one that you may fall into with little thought. It begins with a familiar feeling of dread that begins to hang around. It might start weeks before the dinner, but by the days just prior, it becomes your ever-constant companion.

This response would see you muddle your way through the event, waiting with anxiety to hear if she is, in fact, pregnant. If it is the case, you are likely to feel overwhelming envy, silently withdrawing under a brave face.

This option leaves you feeling anything but calm. Feelings of dread, sadness or resentment can be destructive to both your body and your peace of mind. Dread is certainly the least desirable response to this situation.

### ii) Make a conscious decision not to attend.

One thing needs to be very clear when we discuss this option—this is *not* a cop-out. Depending on your relationship with your family and how much they know about your fertility challenges, you could either explain why you prefer not to be there, or simply find a reason to miss the dinner.

In *Conquering Infertility*, Dr. Alice Domar supports the idea of not putting yourself in a situation that will cause you emotional grief. She refers to this practice as "selective avoidance," encouraging you to steer away from events that will cause you pain.

> Consider this an official prescription: From now on, you don't have to go to baby showers. There, don't you feel better already?[4]

Deciding not to attend the dinner is a strategy that will protect your personal energy, at least in the short term. The main disadvantage, of course, is that it is impractical to avoid your family indefinitely. Chances are very good that you need their love and support in general, and not just because you are trying to become pregnant.

If you choose this option, you may have to find some sort of balance in which you avoid only the events that you know will be the most difficult. While this response is an improvement to dread, there is another option that will serve you better.

---

[4] Dr. Alice Domar, *Conquering Infertility*. (New York: Viking Penguin, 2002), p. 128.

### iii) Detach, detach, detach.

This third option can take much more effort, but it is almost guaranteed to be the most rewarding in the long run. It involves a process of letting go, where you can lessen your attachment to your cousin's news.

By learning to detach yourself, you will be able to reframe the situation entirely. In essence, you will learn to protect yourself by separating slightly from your social surroundings. As you practice this process of letting go, you may be surprised to find how easy it is to let uncomfortable events bounce off of you.

As a start, try the following:

~ Find something (anything) that you are looking forward to about the evening—getting to know your brother's new girlfriend, tasting your aunt's wonderful apple pie or spending a bit of time with your dad.

You name it, if you can genuinely look forward to something about the night, it will make a real difference. Whenever you think of the event, focus on your 'moments' with as much enthusiasm as you can.

Over time, you will likely begin to feel that your cousin's news is not the *only* thing that matters. In fact, it is just one part of the evening.

~ Think about the fact that it's not *their* baby that you want. In fact, their baby has nothing to do with yours. See how far you can separate their baby from your experience in your mind. Try phrases such as:

*Oh well, I didn't want our babies to be the same age anyway.*

*It will be nice for our child to have an older cousin.*

These phrases will be different for each of us. The trick in finding the most useful phrases is to make them personal and believable.

~ Put on a performance. You got it—dust off your acting skills for a good cause. Pretend for the evening that you are not even trying to have children. Yes, it may be hard at times, but you may just be able to convince yourself enough to help.

With these efforts, you may be surprised how easily you can change your view of the situation. Ideally, you will be able to see your cousin's news as just another part of the night, one that you give about the same weight as you would if she were to announce that she was changing jobs.

This reaction to the night is clearly the best for your personal energy, your sense of self and your ability to cope in the long run. As you can imagine, detaching takes plenty of practice. Certainly, some events will be more difficult to handle than others, but the more you can separate yourself from your environment when you need to, the easier it will become to do so.

## Keep At It

Learning to identify your personal triggers is sure to be a work in progress. There will be plenty of times that a trigger event evolves quickly around you, when you suddenly feel uncomfortable or caught off-guard. In order to get through these situations in a way that preserves your sense of calm, a conscious effort is required.

My own journey brought me headlong into the realization that I desperately needed a set of skills for dealing with unwelcome situations. The night of this realization had little that would have been outstanding or uncomfortable to anyone else. From my perspective, however, it became troublesome in a hurry.

It was just after our second IVF cycle had failed, after a summer in which seven of my friends and family members had given birth. I felt extremely introverted. I was still very tender from the sense of loss; I could only see emptiness, doubt and sadness. More than anything, I wanted to be alone.

On this particular night, after two days of steady crying, we had long-standing plans to have dinner with friends. I cried for most of the 45-minute drive to their home.

Our hosts were a wonderful, kind couple. They had two young girls who were beautiful and fun to be around. I knew, at the very least, that our friends were wondering when we were going to have kids. I didn't know if they would ask us about this or not, but I knew that if they did, there was a good chance that I could fall onto the floor in a heaping pile of tears.

Paul was suitably nervous about how the night might unfold, yet felt helpless to make it any better. As we pulled into our friends' driveway, I was barely hanging on. I knew that my eyes revealed all that I had experienced in the last 48 hours.

There was no time for fussing, however, as it was time to get out of the car. I took a deep breath and looked up to see something very promising. There appeared to be another couple arriving at the door. Ah ha! A buffer! Less questions for us and more general conversation—perfect.

As we made our introductions in the front foyer, a sense of relief began to flow through my body. Maybe this dinner would be just the sort of distraction that I needed—a few hours of talking about something other than IVF or babies. Maybe there would even be a few moments of laughter.

What I didn't realize, however, was that the other couple had brought along a special little package. He was tucked around the corner, not making a noise. It was their beautiful four month-old son.

Almost immediately, I was flooded with intense emotions and rapid thoughts:

~ *He's beautiful—how wonderful to be around him.*
~ *You've got to be kidding me…how is this fair?*
~ *What if I burst into tears? Will we have to leave?*
~ *Is the night going to be filled with cooing and baby talk?*

And, of course, the most important question:

~ *Can I handle this?*

Although it was a little touch-and-go at moments throughout the night, I found that the resounding answer to this last question was "yes." I left the evening feeling still cautious, but with gratitude. Somehow, I had been able to detach myself enough to get through the night with some degree of enjoyment.

That evening taught me an important lesson. I realized that I couldn't expect social situations to be forgiving or easy. In order to look out for myself, I needed a set of skills to deal with unwelcome moments, comments or times.

I found myself taking deep breaths through the night. I also tried to smile as much as possible, as it felt like a natural release. More than anything, I believe it was my willingness to detach from the situation, to separate my longing for a baby from the people around me, that saved me from unbearable pain or an awkward explosion of tears.

Every woman going through IVF has her own, similar story. Many have stories far more trying than mine. You may be able to recall moments when you mentally drop to your knees and appeal to whichever god or spirit you call your own to ask:

**Is this real? Do you really expect me to handle this?**

When a trigger event evolves around you, it can be a distinct challenge to maintain a sense of calm. As you gain experience with detachment, however, it will become easier to manage difficult situations. You are sure to find your own way to get through these events; eventually you will be able to distance yourself enough so that they are no longer as challenging.

## Create Deliberate Distractions

Sometimes, the best way to edit the world around you is to indulge in distraction. Unlike relaxation techniques, which generally work best in a specific location and with enough time to indulge yourself, distraction techniques can be used any time, anywhere.

Deliberate distractions are based on the notion that no matter how your journey to parenthood unfolds, no matter how frustrating it is at times, you still have a tremendous capacity to feel good. There is so much more to you than your fertility struggle. You have plenty of reasons to be proud of yourself and grateful for all that you have.

Here are some simple tools to help you get started. Once you begin to practice distractions, you are sure to come up with specific techniques which work for you.

## Make Great Plans

As every woman going through IVF knows, at the very heart of fertility treatment is a schedule. Your days, evenings and weekends are all affected by the schedule of your fertility drugs and procedures. Once you have made room for work and social obligations, there can be precious little time left for you.

Whether you are in the middle of an IVF cycle, or are waiting for one to begin, the key to this distraction is to recognize how under-scheduled you likely are in time for yourself. The fix here is simple, but not something that always comes to mind easily: make great, fantastic plans just for you.

Your plans, big or small, should include things that you will truly look forward to and enjoy. This is not a guilt-laden dinner with friends because it is 'your turn' to have them over, but plans that will make you laugh and lose yourself for a while.

I met Susan online, just as I was starting to realize that I needed a plan to put myself first. Susan was pregnant from her third attempt at IVF and understood exactly what I was feeling.

> I finally 'got it' some time after I learned that cycle #2 was a bust. I realized that I was the only one that could make myself feel better about things. I needed to get happy, to drop guilt towards others and to make plans just for me.
>
> —SUSAN, 39

Think about what makes you truly happy or content. Perhaps it is curling up on the couch to watch your favorite show. Maybe it is going on your own to a favorite spot, taking your dog for a long walk, or catching up with a good friend (who won't ask about babies).

Personally, I had to give this some real thought. Things like shopping, which might be a good distraction for others, never really managed to make me happy. Going out for girls' nights seemed to be a thing of the past, both for me and for my friends with kids.

In the end, I gravitated towards activities that were quiet or provided me with some time alone. I loved the opportunity to go for coffee or breakfast with my girlfriends. I also grew to love my relaxation sessions and yoga classes.

Moments that you truly enjoy have a way of distracting you completely. They are healthy and are usually consuming, leaving little room for negative thoughts to come creeping in. Make great plans as often as you can.

## Laugh Again

Have you ever noticed that when you laugh—really, truly laugh—that it is hard to think about much other than what's got you going? True laughter has a way of bringing us an inner sense of contentedness. It allows us to block out everything and to 'get back to ourselves.'

A good laugh has well-documented medical benefits, as well. Laughter is known to have an incredible, restorative power. It has been shown to lower blood pressure, increase muscle flexion and trigger the release of endorphins, our natural 'feel good' chemicals. There are plenty of benefits for our immune systems and stress levels, as well.

Of course, true laughter may seem like a distant memory when you're in the middle of a frustrating fertility struggle. There is often just too much going on, too much stress and too much anxiety to truly indulge in laughter. Naturally, this is when you need a good laugh the most.

Once you are aware of how important it is to laugh, you are more likely to find opportunities to do so. When you start looking, you may be surprised to find how readily they are available.

Start by renting funny movies, reading something that will make you smile, spending more time chatting to your co-worker who always makes you laugh.

Get creative if you need to, but trust that the more you can laugh, the better you will feel, and the more positive your physical condition will be.

## Indulge in Praise

Praise is something that is usually easy and enjoyable to give. As women, it is also something that we most often reserve for others. When is the last time that you complimented yourself? How often do you really, truly feel good about yourself and tell yourself so?

For many women, the idea of self-praise will be so foreign that it will sound silly or overly indulgent. It can have a lasting, powerful effect in your life, however, if you allow yourself permission to be proud.

Examples of self-praise include thoughts such as:

~ *I think I handled that situation well.*
~ *I'm proud of the work that I put into that project.*
~ *I have a lot of compassion for others.*

I first came across the idea of self-praise when I looked into the Law of Attraction, a body of thought that holds that you can draw your desires into your life with focused, positive attention. Naturally, I was intrigued by this concept and wondered if it could apply to my fertility situation.

I found that it was truly helpful. Perhaps most important, it helped me to understand the strength of my personal energy. The Law of Attraction holds that self-praise is a forgiving, positive exercise that allows you to elevate your personal energy.

When I decided to give self-praise a shot, I chose to focus on something

**What You Can Do!**
To learn more about the Law of Attraction, consider the works of Michael Losier, Esther and Jerry Hicks or Lynn Grabhorn.

that I knew was going well: work. I could always muster a positive thought about something I had achieved or a situation that I handled well. Over time, I admitted that there were other things that I did well: finding great friends, treating others with compassion and more.

I met Sylvia when she was between cycles. I noticed that she was remarkably calm and positive about her situation and wondered if she might be putting on a brave face. Over time, I realized that she really was as content as she appeared.

When I asked her how she kept so positive, she described the process of using self-praise:

> It's not always easy. There are times that I'm basically inconsolable. Generally though, when I do start to feel down, I try to focus on my 'other' life—you know, the part where things are actually going right! It just helps me to realize that my whole life is not defined by IVF.
> —SYLVIA, 36

To get started with your own list of praise, try finding moments or thoughts when you truly feel genuine self-appreciation. Your efforts shouldn't feel over-done or put-on, but somehow refreshing and real.

## A Level Result

Learning how to edit the world around you should be empowering. Whether you are identifying your personal trigger events, choosing how to respond to an awkward situation or deliberately distracting yourself for a moment of escape, you are taking action to preserve your peace of mind.

Once you give yourself permission to separate yourself in these ways, you will likely start to level out your emotions. Over time, it will get easier to find true joy in things outside of your fertility journey.

As you do so, you will become more and more deliberate with your energy. You may be surprised to find how little steps begin to generate subtle changes in how you view IVF and the rest of the world.

Next, we will look at a very important list. It has nothing to do with your regular 'to-dos'. It is about finding positive, proactive things that you can do to put yourself first through IVF. By indulging in these simple activities, you are sure to improve your personal energy and your odds of IVF success.

# CHAPTER NINE
# Creating Your New To-Do List

Because it is always empowering to take action through a difficult situation, doing something positive—no matter how small—is an important part of nurturing yourself through IVF. In this chapter, we will look at several ways that you can take positive action before and during a cycle.

Your new To-Do List includes the following:

- ~ Find Great Support
- ~ Write it Down
- ~ Explore Advantages Through Diet
- ~ Do Your Own Research
- ~ Lose Your Superstitions
- ~ Have a Plan
- ~ Lean on Your Clinic
- ~ Practice Your Nurturing

You may be surprised by some of the suggestions found here. Keep in mind that they can all improve your odds of success by helping to level out your energy, to inject positive energy into your daily life and to help preserve your sense of self through it all.

## Find Great Support

Evidence shows that support groups can help to reduce some of the most common emotional struggles faced by women going through IVF: anxiety, depression and feelings of isolation. The only trick, it seems, is finding the right kind of support for you.

Personally, I found that a combination of online and face-to-face support worked best for me. I liked the immediate feedback of an online environment, but found that connecting with women in person felt natural and rewarding.

I've met several women who prefer the face-to-face group environment best of all. Some prefer the structure of a regular meeting time, some prefer personal conversations to an online environment and others simply like to be able to look around the room to feel a true connection with others.

Whether you prefer to connect online or in person, it is important to find a group in which you find the understanding and encouragement that you need. Even if you connect with one other woman who knows just what you are going through, you will be at a great advantage.

"Appendix One: A Few Great Resources" offers a list of support resources. I encourage you to try a variety of groups and environments. You will know when you have found a support group that seems to fit.

## Write it Down

Although I had never kept a journal, I found that writing down my thoughts and feelings during my last cycle was the single most valuable tool for improving my experience through IVF. I am confident that this can help you, as well.

I started to keep a journal on the recommendation of Dr. Terry Willard in his book, *Mind-Body Harmony, How to Resist and Recover From Auto-Immune Diseases*. Dr. Willard suggests that using a release such as journal-keeping is an important way to let go of the "emotional roughage," or unhealthy feelings, that we pick up in our daily lives.

He claims that some of the healthiest people develop some of the most difficult health issues, and that many of these people are emotionally sensitive, with a perfectionist streak. Sensitive people tend to hold on to emotions in a way that creates a low-grade, unhealthy level of stress.

> I noticed that patients who developed autoimmune issues were often living only in their heads.... Worry, tension, stress and emotional crisis occupied their minds and yet they seemed oblivious to the reality that their being was depositing this stress in the physical body.[5]

Dr. Willard's book was a wake-up call for me. At the time, I was only wondering if immune issues were part of my fertility challenges. Even so, his description of generally healthy patients who are emotionally sensitive and slightly perfectionist was entirely familiar. It not only described me, but also many of the women that I had met going through IVF.

---

[5] Dr. Terry Willard, *Mind-Body Harmony*. (Toronto: Sarasota Press, 2002), pp. 29–30.

There is plenty of other support for the health benefits of keeping a journal, as well. A recent four-month study published in the *Journal of the American Medical Association* found that writing down details about particularly stressful events could improve the health of patients who suffer from the chronic conditions such as asthma and arthritis.

With nothing to lose, I decided to give journal-keeping a try. I decided that my train ride to work could act as my dedicated time and place for journal entries. I made a promise to myself that I wouldn't put pressure on the amount of time that I spent writing, nor the length of each entry made.

What I wrote surprised me. It was everything. It was details about injections, feelings about comments made to me at work, thoughts about the distant future, fears about the near future and more. I just really let everything go. I took comfort knowing that I could repeat my frustrations and worries as often as I wanted and that nobody would read it.

The results were almost immediate. Suddenly, I found myself looking forward to my journal sessions. It was a very short, daily appointment with myself that left me feeling balanced and just simply better. I was truly amazed how something so seemingly small could make such a difference.

## Explore Advantages Through Diet

Although I hesitate to make any mention of diet in a book that is written for women, I think this point is well worth covering. Don't worry, I'm not going to suggest that you limit caffeine or avoid alcohol—we can leave the clearly obvious to the popular magazines.

What you want to know is, "Is there something, through diet, that I can do to help myself?" The answer, though not entirely straightforward, seems to be "probably, yes." Depending on the nature of your diagnosis, there may be plenty that you can do.

Although I am not a nutritionist or any sort of specialist with respect to diet and fertility, I do know that exploring this subject gave me a much-needed sense of empower-ment. I considered diet suggestions made by my RE, by naturopaths, and by those found in Chinese medicine.

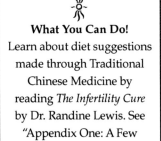

**What You Can Do!**
Learn about diet suggestions made through Traditional Chinese Medicine by reading *The Infertility Cure* by Dr. Randine Lewis. See "Appendix One: A Few Great Resources."

I ended up following a diet that matched my diagnosis through Chinese medicine. In order to help balance my body and help it heal from endometriosis, for example, I decided to avoid dairy and all foods that had been hormonally treated.

In order to help improve my blood circulation, I added things such as peppermint tea, onions and lemons. In order to help balance my immune system, I tried to stay away from wheat products.

There were many more changes, but once I had a good understanding of the diet itself, it was fairly easy to work into my life. I liked that there was something proactive that I could do *right away* and *throughout the day* to improve the conditions of my body. Whether I was choosing to avoid or add particular foods, I felt empowered every time that I made a decision around my diet.

I am confident that if you choose to explore advantages that may be available through diet, that you will feel equally empowered. You may need to explore several suggested diets in order to find one that feels right to you. Trust your instinct and listen to your body—you are sure to find a diet that fits your diagnosis and your comfort level.

## Do Your Own Research

As we've seen, one of the most frustrating aspects of going through IVF is feeling an absence of control. You do what your doctors tell you, plain and simple. You feel unlike yourself as hormones do their work. Your schedule and lifestyle are clearly altered without your input.

One of the best ways to regain a sense of control is to do your own research. This is not to say that you should become an expert in reproductive endocrinology, or that you should question every decision made by your doctors.

Your research might start with a second or third opinion. You may begin to read more about your diagnosis and seek the support of others in the same situation. Don't be afraid to ask questions, even if you think that you should know the answer. Perhaps the best place to get started with this sort of research is the Internet.

Chances are, you have already done some exploration online, and have been able to find women who share your diagnosis and/or feelings. In "Appendix One: A Few Great Resources," you will find a list of helpful web sites that feature bulletin boards, online chats and clinic-specific information. These are terrific places to share and learn.

It was through an online forum called Fertile Thoughts (www.fertilethoughts.com), that I first met Tanya, a woman who pointed me in the right direction to explore my immune issues. With her guidance, I learned how to send my blood to be tested for specific antibodies, and how to find the right doctor to treat me.

Given that it was my first cycle with treatment for my immune system (intravenous immunoglobulin—IVIG) that led to a successful pregnancy, I am enormously grateful that I met Tanya online. I am convinced that it was an important part of my success. I am thankful that Tanya was so generous with her information and had a willingness to help others.

Just a word of caution while exploring on the Internet: be careful. First, you need to consider the credibility of the information you receive. As you are sure to find conflicting information, try not to become overwhelmed or frustrated. Simply trust your instinct and check your facts with your doctor.

I would also advise you to be careful not to fall into the negative thoughts or energy of others online. When you start to meet other women going through IVF, you are sure to find those who are negative or so skeptical that their Internet postings leave you feeling slightly down.

This is not to say that you should only read happy, perky postings, but take notice of how you feel after your online experiences. Try to gravitate towards a group of women who are more positive, supportive and helpful. Try to find those who are more in line with where you want to be.

Whichever route makes you more comfortable, doing your own research can be an important part of nurturing yourself through IVF. It can give you self-confidence when you need it most; it can give you a sense of empowerment when it feels like your only other option is to wait.

## Lose Your Superstitions

As I met more and more women going through IVF, I realized that there were plenty that shared a bad habit of mine. I had become superstitious. It was ridiculous and offered no value to my experience, but I would regularly catch myself playing games of chance.

The outcome of random events, in my mind, was always whether or not I would become pregnant. In effect, I was giving away even more control by allowing these acts of chance to affect my mood and sense of optimism. Throughout my first cycle, I would catch myself with thoughts such as:

~ *If I beat that car to the next stoplight, I will get a positive pregnancy test.*
~ *If I see any babies on the way to the clinic today, it will be positive.*
~ *If the elevator arrives with nobody on it, it will be positive.*

It went on and on. I hardly knew that I was doing it until a friend remarked on her views of superstition.

> I used to be superstitious, but after I got a negative last time, I'm not anymore. Why bother?
> —JENNY, 34

I knew right away that Jenny was right. Superstition had no positive place in my mind. The only thing it accomplished was to make me more nervous than I might have been. In hindsight, I can see that it was a useless activity that only contributed to a turbulent pattern of personal energy.

With my second and third cycles, I worked to catch my superstitious thoughts. It did take some work, but I vowed to be vigilant. Thankfully, the benefits were immediate. As soon as I released my superstitions, I felt relieved, free and more relaxed.

If superstitions are part of your experience through IVF, consider letting them go. If you can truly believe that they serve no purpose, and in fact can bring you more anxiety, it will be easy to turn them off. You will likely feel that you have regained some degree of control.

## Have a Plan

Among the many women that I met going through IVF, I found a recurring personality trait: many of us are incurable planners. If you are a planner yourself, you know just what this means. You like lists, you like an organized approach to your day and you feel that somehow, life just works better with a plan.

Naturally, a fertility struggle is one of the most frustrating experiences for a planner to encounter. Even within the structure of an IVF cycle, there are enough variables and unknowns that make it difficult to plan around. You will most likely find that your clinic is hesitant to talk about 'next steps' until they know the outcome of a given test or cycle.

This is where your plan comes in. If you consider yourself to be a planner, try to embrace this characteristic. It is okay to want to have a plan. If you are not a planner by nature, you may find it both reassuring and empowering to build a plan while you are in any sort of waiting period through IVF.

As you start to map out your own direction, write down questions that you may want to ask your RE at your next visit. If you are interested in a second or third opinion, consider who you might contact. Find women online who may already know about clinics, procedures or options that may interest you. Keeping a broad perspective about what might work for you can save you from feeling that your current path is the only option available.

I met Christie when she was in the middle of a two-week wait. Based on the assessment of the single embryo that she had transferred, she was quite sure that the cycle hadn't worked. Rather than building up a false sense of hope, she simply wanted to move on with a plan.

> **I feel like I'm totally in limbo. My clinic won't even talk about what's next until a follow-up appointment, which will probably be three weeks after my (pregnancy) test. I want to do something right now—this waiting is killing me.**
>
> —CHRISTIE, 36

**What You Can Do!**
To find a brief second opinion on a basic question, try going online to one of the many bulletin boards answered by doctors. See "Appendix One," under 'Online Support and Information.'

When I spoke to Christie three days later, she felt much better. She still didn't know the outcome of her cycle, but she had booked an appointment for a second opinion and had done some research on egg donation. She didn't know which way she would go next time, but she felt much better knowing that she and her husband had taken things into their own hands.

Having your own plan allows you the freedom to explore your options, and provides a sense of control that you may be craving. Although you can't know how things will unfold, you may come up with a healthy 'if-then' approach.

~ *If this doesn't work, then we'll ask to try a different protocol.*

~ *If our doctor isn't willing to try something different next time, then we'll seek out a second opinion.*

## Lean on Your Clinic

One of the most common things that I heard from women going through IVF was how difficult and lonely they found the waiting periods within a cycle. Because clinic staff members need to communicate with dozens of women every day, their conversations with individuals are naturally quite short. These brief exchanges can leave you wanting more.

Catherine, who I met through a friend, wanted much more from her clinic. Her retrieval had produced a disappointing number of eggs, and very few had fertilized. She was restlessly waiting to hear further news on her embryos.

> They didn't say much—only that just three of them fertilized and that there might be a problem with my eggs. I was in shock. I got off the phone and thought of all the questions that I should have asked.
>
> —CATHERINE, 33

This is a common interaction that can leave you feeling powerless. If you are surprised by your clinic's news, you may tune out entirely and miss details that you might wonder about later.

Part of nurturing yourself through IVF includes taking an active role in communicating with your clinic. If you are waiting for a phone call, write down questions that you might have ahead of time. Ask if there is a number where you can call back with any questions.

Let your clinic staff know if you are in pain, if you have questions about your health or if you feel that you are struggling emotionally. Your clinic is there to help and can be a terrific resource for helping you through the whole experience.

Personally, I have been grateful for the clinic interactions that I have had. The nurses have always welcomed questions and have been very supportive.

I know that this is not the relationship that all women have with their clinics, however. If you feel resistance from your clinic, insist that they spend the time to answer your questions. This is an emotional experience and a significant investment. You deserve patient, kind and helpful service.

## Practice Your Nurturing

Nurturing is something that we have touched upon throughout this book. Self-nurturing can be an important way of maximizing your health and your peace of mind. Because it sometimes helps to have a simple exercise to get started, you may want to practice with the following.

Without a doubt, you know that you will love and nurture your children. Imagine one of your future children going through a challenging emotional period. What would you say to him or her?

Perhaps you would use supportive phrases such as:

~ *Hey kiddo, you're going to get there. You're doing a great job.*
~ *You're stronger than you know. You'll get through this.*
~ *It's going to be okay. Keep going—it's all going to work out.*

These nurturing thoughts are enormously powerful. Try saying them out loud and see how you feel. We all have moments and times when we need to know that it's all going to be okay. You deserve to hear these thoughts every day from the most important voice in your life—your own.

Although it is easy to imagine offering such tenderness to future children, it might seem silly or self-indulgent to use the same phrases for yourself. Self-nurturing is not something that we do naturally—it can take a good deal of practice. To help yourself get started, try writing down your own phrases and refer to them when you have some time to yourself.

## Control Regained

As we've seen over and over, it is much easier to do something, to take action through an IVF cycle, than to let it simply unfold before you. Your new To-Do list should help you to do just that. It is about finding simple, practical things that allow you to feel more in control of your daily life.

We have looked at just a few of the ways that you can consciously improve your state of mind through IVF. You will certainly discover more of your own tools and techniques if you are open to finding them. You may be surprised to find just how quickly a bit of control helps you to feel more positive and deliberate with your energy.

Next, I would like to offer some simple encouragement. You are at a difficult passage in your life, doing all that you can to become a mother. If you need to start with small steps to improve your journey through IVF, trust that every effort you make is helpful. Trust your instinct as you go. You can do this, and you deserve to hear as much encouragement as possible.

# CHAPTER TEN

# You Can Do This

THROUGHOUT THIS BOOK, we've looked at both practical tools and mental strategies to help nurture yourself through IVF. Here, I would like to offer you some heartfelt encouragement from someone who understands. You have more strength than you realize, you have tremendous love for your future children and you can do this.

For some reason, IVF has become part of your life experience. Although it is not the way any one of us would have imagined becoming a parent from the outset, it is where you and I, and many others, have landed.

If you are just starting an IVF journey, you've seen that many decisions lie before you. Some are about clinics, doctors and medical procedures. Others concern logistics—how you will weave IVF into your work and social life. I maintain, however, that the most important decisions are those concerning *you*. How will you treat yourself through this time? Will you find ways to put yourself first? How can you feel genuinely happy again? How can you begin to believe that no matter what happens, you're going to be okay?

## Believing Before Seeing

An important part of putting yourself first is learning how to truly believe. Although we are inclined to associate believing with religion or spirituality, it can be thought of in a much broader context, as well. You need to believe in yourself, believe in the future and believe that somehow, some way, you will become a parent.

I started writing this book when I was between IVF cycles. Part of the reason I felt compelled to do so was simply an observation of the many women that I met through my travels. I could see that we had a lot of feelings and emotions in common, and that most of us could benefit from the principles of mind-body healing and an understanding of our personal energy.

Just as compelling, was an unshakable belief that my husband and I would somehow become parents. I just had a feeling that it might be helpful to share our experience with others. I mentioned earlier that I believe that I was meant to experience all that IVF entails; this sort of belief is forgiving, strengthening and healing. I hope that you are eventually able to feel the same way.

By any definition, belief is about trust. Whether you are believing in a higher power or in your own ability to cope through this time, it is a simultaneous sense of letting go and accepting. It allows you to get to your destination mentally, long before it becomes a reality.

The benefit of believing as you go through IVF is that your body and mind begin to open up. They can work in incredible ways to help maximize your physical conditions and improve your odds of success, even without conscious effort.

**What You Can Do!**
For inspiration on the power of your thoughts and energy, consider reading the works of Wayne W. Dyer, including *You'll See It When You Believe It.*

More than just believing that you will one day hold your baby in your arms, you *must* believe that you deserve to be happy. If you can truly embrace the notion that you deserve happiness, it will find you. This is a self-fulfilling prophecy that is fueled by your positive energy and your willingness to trust that things will work out for the best.

I know that believing through an IVF cycle can be hard, especially when you've experienced negative results in the past. I encourage you to read broadly on the subject of believing, however, and to realize that you are only part way through your journey. You don't yet know what the end destination will be. Believe in your ability to cope as you go, and trust that your miracles are coming.

## Rising Up

As we saw early in this book, it is natural and even healthy to fall down once in a while through your IVF experience. Part of what helps you to get up when you've fallen is your deep-rooted strength. Your desire to have a baby has given you the patience and perseverance to even *get* to an IVF cycle. I hope that you can take pride in your strength and focus.

An IVF cycle is not for the faint of heart. It takes planning, perseverance, courage and commitment. It is manageable, but not easy; tolerable, but at times torturous. You should be proud of yourself and your strength.

Trust that you are doing everything in your power to have success with IVF. Be gentle and forgiving with yourself. Know that with your focus and energy, and with love for yourself, you can do this.

# CHAPTER ELEVEN
## Conclusion

As I complete the final edits for this book, I am in a very familiar position: I am preparing to begin a frozen cycle. I cannot pretend to have the same level of anxiety as I did before my daughter arrived, but I am surprised to find negative feelings lurking close by.

I have the sense that doubt, fear and many other unpleasant feelings are waiting for me, should I choose to let them wreak havoc with my personal energy.

I am reminded that this is a difficult, personal journey and that it is natural to feel hope, fear, doubt and excitement, often all at once. I know that I will do well to heed my own advice—to make a steady effort to remain calm and positive. I do trust that even the smallest effort will help.

I hope that you have been able to find some comfort and encouragement in the pages of this book. I hope that you will embrace the ideas behind the mind-body connection and will be open to making it work for you. Finally, I hope that you begin to see your IVF experience differently. You deserve to focus on *yourself*, rather than the expectations that the rest of the world may have of you.

## Your Best Results

Have patience with yourself as you begin to make the changes suggested throughout this book. It can take time to fall into a routine that incorporates time for yourself. It can take a while to understand and appreciate how your personal energy affects your body.

Your best results through IVF will unfold when you are kind to yourself and are willing to keep an open mind. I am confident that you can find your own best path through this journey. It is a long, difficult road to parenthood, but you have the power to make the most of it. Trust in yourself and know that no matter what happens, you're going to be okay.

# APPENDIX ONE

# A Few Great Resources

THROUGH MY OWN JOURNEY, and with the help of the many women that I've met, I have learned of some excellent resources to help make IVF a little easier to navigate and handle. Consider exploring these groups, places and products to help you make the most of your experience.

Please note that the web links provided are subject to change over time.

## Support Groups

We've seen the undeniable benefits provided by the right kind of support group. As you look for one that best suits your needs, keep in mind that you can explore several options before settling into one group.

Here are a few places to start your search:

### Your clinic

Many clinics have peer support groups or 'cycle buddy'

programs, through which you can meet other women going through IVF. The advantage of this kind of support is that it is local, it is often face-to-face, and you are more likely to have similar kinds of experiences and drug protocols.

If you do happen to meet someone who is cycling at the same time as you, it is very helpful to see a smiling, friendly face in the clinic waiting room. This kind of support feels very real, immediate and personal. Having a local cycle buddy can definitely improve your experience through IVF.

### Resolve

Resolve is a U.S.-based organization with more than 50 local chapters available nationwide. If you are interested in support and do not live near one of the local chapters, Resolve has an informal member-to-member medical contact system that may be available to you.

(www.resolve.org)

### American Fertility Association (AFA)

The AFA offers a wide range of support groups, including those based on specific interests such as 'Orthodox Jewish Issues', 'Secondary Infertility', 'Are You Ready to Adopt?' and many more.

(www.theafa.org)

### Infertility Awareness Association of Canada (IAAC)

The IAAC offers support groups across the country, from British Columbia to Prince Edward Island.

(www.iaac.ca)

**Other**

You may also be able to find local 'face-to-face' support groups that are not associated with a national organization. Try doing an Internet search with the name of your town or city along with keywords such as "support group," "infertility" or "IVF."

## Online Support and Information

As mentioned earlier, the Internet can be an excellent place to conduct research and find support. You can very likely find women online who share your diagnosis, those who are cycling at the same time as you, those who are in your city/town or even those who are receiving treatment at your clinic.

Online support can be terrific, as you can connect with others whenever you feel like logging on. You can participate anonymously if you wish, and you can easily search for historical chats or conversations that may help you.

Be warned that it is easy to become misguided or overwhelmed with information that you find on the Internet. Trust your instinct as you go and be sure to check your findings with your doctor.

### Bulletin Boards

Bulletin boards, also known as forums, discussion boards or 'blogs' (for web logs), can be an excellent resource for women going through IVF. You can usually browse by subject area, and can read through 'threads' or online conversations.

Bulletin boards are particularly useful if you have a specific question that you would like to have answered.

Typically, you would start a new thread or conversation with your question. Usually within a day or two, someone will respond.

I liked using bulletin boards because you can explore entire conversations on a subject, even if you weren't 'there' when it took place. A few places to find bulletin boards include:

~ IVF Connections
  (www.ivfconnections.com)

~ Fertile Thoughts
  (www.fertilethoughts.com)

~ INCIID—The InterNational Council on Infertility
  Information Dissemination
  (www.inciid.org—look for 'Forums')

~ Resolve—The National Infertility Association
  (www.resolve.org—look for 'Bulletin Board')

~ American Fertility Association
  (www.theafa.org—look for 'Message Boards')

~ IVF-Infertility.com
  (www.ivf-infertility.com—look for 'Message Board')

~ Infertility Central.com
  (www.fertilityforums.com)

**Doctor Response Boards**

The following sites offer bulletin boards on which doctors or specialists respond directly to questions from site visitors.

~ INCIID
(www.inciid.org—look for 'Ask an Expert' under 'Forums')

~ SIRM—Sher Institutes for Reproductive Medicine
(www.haveababy.com—look for 'Discussion and Communication')

~ Shady Grove Fertility
(www.shadygrovefertility.com—look for 'Ask an Expert')

~ IRMS—The Institute for Reproductive Medicine and Science of St. Barnabas
(www.sbivf.com—look for 'Message Board')

~ Huntington Reproductive Center
(www.havingbabies.com—look for 'Ask Our Doctors')

If you are interested in direct physician feedback, there are plenty of other clinics that offer this service online, as well.

Of course, it is difficult for the responding doctors to go into too much detail about your situation without assessing you themselves, but this type of resource can be very helpful for finding answers or opinions on brief questions.

**Online Chats**

Online chats are terrific places to share and learn. Web sites that offer chats generally have a doctor or an expert available to help answer questions. Chats take place at a specific time and you have the option to participate anonymously.

In my experience, the only down-side to chats is that by their very nature, they are rapid. Doctors are often fielding several questions at once, so they need to be brief in their answers. Naturally, for a subject as complex as infertility, this can leave you wanting more.

When you participate in an online chat, have your questions ready ahead of time, ask one question at a time and be willing to ask your question in a different way if you don't receive the type of answer that you are hoping for.

Look for chat 'transcripts' for a record of previous sessions. Although you won't necessarily have your questions answered directly, they can be a valuable source of information.

~ INCIID
  (www.inciid.org—look for 'Chat')

~ Resolve—The National Infertility Association
  (www.resolve.org—look for 'Online Chat')

~ SIRM—Sher Institutes for Reproductive Medicine
  (www.haveababy.com—look for 'Chat With Infertility Experts'
  or 'Live Chat Events')

**Webinars**
Webinars are essentially online seminars. Like live chats, they take place at a specific time and generally feature a doctor or specialist speaker. Although it depends on the technology used, you will usually have the opportunity to ask questions at the end.

Generally speaking, however, a webinar is more about receiving the information presented than it is about asking your specific questions. Be patient when you are viewing a webinar for the first time—it sometimes takes a few minutes to load the presentation and audio.

Look for fertility clinics that host their own webinars as educational tools. They allow clinics to promote their expertise, and allow you to interact from the comfort of your home.

~ INCIID
(www.inciid.org)

## Other Online Resources

~ American Society for Reproductive Medicine
(www.asrm.org)

~ Centre for Journal Therapy
(www.journaltherapy.com)

~ The Fertile Soul
(www.thefertilesoul.com)

~ Fertility Friends (UK)
(www.fertilityfriends.co.uk)

~ Fertility Network
(www.fertilitynetwork.com)

~ Infertility Awareness Association of Canada
(www.iaac.ca)

~ Infertility Network (Canada)
(www.infertilitynetwork.org)

~ IVF.net
(www.ivf.net)

~ Mind | Body Institute for Infertility (Los Angeles)
www.mindbodyinfertility.com)

~ Mind Body Medical Institute
(www.mbmi.org)

~ Mind-Body Medicine Canada
(www.mindbodycan.com)

~ Mind-Body-Fertility (New York and Connecticut)
(www.mind-body-fertility.com)

~ Yoga Journal
(www.yogajournal.com)

## Recordings

As mentioned, I found that my mind was too active through IVF to truly relax without the aid of an audio recording. You will be able to find plenty of relaxation recordings online, but you may also want to see if your local library has any that you can try before buying.

A few of my personal favorites include:

~ *Your Present: A Half-Hour of Peace*
Susie Mantell
(available from www.amazon.com)

This CD offers a wonderful, positive sense of escape. Although it is not specifically about fertility, it is relevant and very helpful.

~ Guided Imagery from Anji Inc.
(www.anjionline.com)

Anji offers CDs for general fertility enhancement, as well as one specifically for IVF patients. On the CD titled

"Imagery and Meditations to Support In-Vitro Fertilization (IVF)," recordings are structured to support you through the different stages of your cycle.

~ *Hypnotherapy for Fertility*
Insight Hypnosis
(www.wendi.com)

This CD is about fertility in general, and not just IVF, but it is different from basic relaxation. I found it quite powerful as a distraction / relaxation tool.

~ *Yoga 4 Fertility*
Brenda Strong
(www.yoga4fertility.com)

~ *Fertility Yoga*
Monica Morell
(www.fertilityoga.com)

## Books

Throughout this book, I've referred to several books that have helped me along the way. Reading is one of the best things that you can do through a fertility struggle. It can provide you with inspiration, new ideas or even a new way to approach your journey. It is helpful to read books that are both related to infertility as well as those that are not.

Here are some of the books that I have found most helpful:

~ *The Infertility Cure: The Ancient Chinese Wellness
Program for Getting Pregnant and Having Healthy Babies*
(Dr. Randine Lewis, 2004).

~ *Conquering Infertility: Dr. Alice Domar's Mind/Body Guide to Enhancing Fertility and Coping with Infertility* (Dr. Alice D. Domar, 2002).

~ *Healing Mind, Healthy Woman: Using the Mind/Body Connection to Manage Stress and Take Control of Your Life* (Dr. Alice D. Domar, 1996).

~ *Mind-Body Harmony: How to Resist and Recover From Auto-Immune Diseases* (Dr. Terry Willard, 2003).

~ *Endometriosis, Infertility & Chinese Medicine: A Laywoman's Guide* (Bob Flaws, 1989).

~ *Excuse Me, Your Life is Waiting: The Astonishing Power of Feelings* (Lynn Grabhorn, 2003)

~ *You'll See It When You Believe It: The Way to Your Personal Transformation* (Wayne W. Dyer, 2001)

# APPENDIX TWO

# One Successful Cycle

As MENTIONED, MY HUSBAND PAUL and I went through three years of testing, surgery and treatment before we had success with IVF. We've gone through three cycles in total: two fresh and one frozen. Here, I will list all of the things that we did for our last cycle, which resulted in a successful pregnancy.

Please keep in mind that I am not a doctor, and that my experience is unique. Your circumstances and diagnosis will require your doctor's opinion and treatment, as well as your research and perseverance.

## Diagnosis

- ~ male factor: low count
- ~ one laparoscopy revealed a mild case of endometriosis, two years before our successful cycle
- ~ small uterine septum

~ Raynaud's Syndrome and results of immune system tests pointed to the fact that I may have an immunological barrier to pregnancy

## Medical Treatment

~ After two unsuccessful cycles at another clinic, we had success with the Markham Fertility Centre (Ontario, Canada), under the care of Dr. Michael Virro.

~ I had been on a two-month dose of Depot Lupron, to treat endometriosis, several months before our cycle began.

~ I had sent my blood for testing at Millenova Immunology Laboratories in Chicago, where the 'Implantation Failure Panel' revealed that I had several elevated antibodies.

~ With Dr. David Clark in Hamilton, Canada I had my immune system treated with Intravenous immunoglobulin (IVIG) and heparin, before my transfer and throughout my pregnancy.

~ We transferred two three-day embryos, and had six others go on to the blastocyst stage, where they were frozen.

## Traditional Chinese Medicine (TCM) Therapies

~ I went to see a doctor of Chinese medicine who specializes in fertility. I received acupuncture sessions for two months prior to the cycle. I also took Chinese herbs for one month prior.

I stopped the herbs before I started any medical treatment for the cycle, as I was cautious about mixing the two therapies. Dr. Virro needed to know what he was working with and I didn't feel that would be the case if I was still taking them.

~ I received acupuncture treatments before and after our embryo transfer. Specific points were treated, according to a 2002 German study that found an increased rate of pregnancy when IVF was complimented with particular acupuncture treatment.

~ I followed a diet specific to my diagnosis and bodily conditions, according to Chinese medicine. Beyond eliminating caffeine and alcohol, I reduced my sugar intake, eliminated dairy, and did my best to reduce the amount of wheat in my diet.

~ Although I thought my conditions (mild endometriosis and possible immune issues) seemed complicated, I found direct, simple diet recommendations in Dr. Randine Lewis' *The Infertility Cure.*

Please note that if you decide to pursue therapies in Chinese medicine, it is strongly recommended by Dr. Lewis and other experts that you deal only with licensed professionals, preferably those that specialize in fertility. Make sure that your RE is aware of any alternative therapy that you receive.

## Lifestyle

~ Although I love the endorphin rush of a good workout, I made a conscious effort to tone down my level of exercise leading up to the cycle. Because my RE had recommended taking things easy, I replaced runs with walks and tried to see this as an overall sense of slowing down to prepare for pregnancy.

~ On the recommendation of a former R
yoga three times a week. I always left
more relaxed than when I went in. I c
time of my egg retrieval.

## Relaxation

~ I experimented with a few forms of relaxation before I
found the ones that made me most comfortable. I liked
using guided sessions with the aid of audio recordings.

I used recordings that were fertility related, but usually
preferred those that were not. My personal favorite was
given to me by a friend, called "Your Present: A Half-
Hour of Peace" by Susie Mantell.

~ I found that I relied on my husband's support to make
regular relaxation possible. Leading up to my cycle, I
would usually do three sessions a week, but as it drew
very close I was doing them every day.

Paul's support for the time required for relaxation was
invaluable. Whether he was taking care of things
around the house or giving up some of our 'together'
time, his support was enormously helpful.

## Journal Keeping

~ As mentioned, I found keeping a journal to be the single most valuable tool in improving my experience
through IVF. I started doing it mostly as an experiment,
to see if it would make a difference. I found that it did
so right away. I was able to part with all sorts of
thoughts and emotions that I might have otherwise
held onto.

I made a point of tucking my small journal into my purse, so that I wouldn't forget it on my way to work. With a 45-minute train ride, I found it easy to pull out my journal and jot a few things down on my way to the office. I would spend 5–10 minutes writing about work, the details of my cycle—anything that was on my mind.

## Believing

~ Belief is such a personal thing. I happen to believe in a God and find that quite comforting. I didn't just pray for a baby—I prayed for the strength to get through this difficult chapter of my life. I know that other people prayed for us too, and for that I am very grateful.

~ As mentioned, I also had an unshakable belief that things would just work out, that IVF would work for us. Call it a hunch, my instinct or a self-fulfilling prophecy, I just knew that if we could persevere, that we would find an answer.

## Instinct

~ I don't want to underestimate the role that my instinct played in our successful cycle. While we all have instinct, it can be difficult to 'hear' it sometimes. Through my last cycle, I let my instinct lead me as much as possible.

Instinct is what led me to seek the opinion of Dr. Virro; it is what led me to pursue immune system testing and treatment, and to compliment my medical treatment with other tools: diet, acupuncture, relaxation and more.

I want to emphasize again that my circumstances and conditions are entirely unique. These practices are simply what worked best for me at the time. I do not suggest that you recreate this entire scenario yourself, but I do hope that it provides you with a few ideas and perhaps the motivation to experiment with ways to improve your own experience through IVF.

# References

"Benefits of Yoga" (n.d.). Retrieved February 1, 2006 from:
http://www.emedicinehealth.com/articles/10795-4.asp

Benson, Herbert, M.D. *The Relaxation Response.* New York:
Harpertorch, 2000.

Berk, Lee S., Dr., and Dr. Stanley Tan. "The Laughter-Immune
Connection: New Discoveries," Humor and Health Journal
(1996): vol. 5, no. 5.

Domar, Alice D., PhD. *Conquering Infertility.* New York: Penguin
Group, 2002.

Dyer, Wayne W. *You'll See It When You Believe It: The Way to Your
Personal Transformation.* New York: Harper Collins, 2001.

Leduc, Marc. "Breathing for Health." Retrieved February 1,
2006 from:
http://www.healingdaily.com/exercise/breathing.htm

Lewis, Randine, PhD. *The Infertility Cure.* New York: Little,
Brown and Company, 2004.

Paulus, et al. "Influence of acupuncture on the pregnancy rate
in patients who undergo assisted reproduction therapy,"
Fertility and Sterility (April, 2002): Vol. 77, No. 4.

Sgovio, Robert. "Conscious Deep Breathing." Retrieved February 1, 2006 from: http://healing.about.com/od/breath work/a/consciousbreath.htm

Smyth, Joshua M, PhD. and Arthur A. Stone, PhD. "Effects of Writing About Stressful Experiences on Symptom Reduction in Patients With Asthma or Rheumatoid Arthritis," Journal of the American Medical Association (April, 1999): Vol. 281 No. 14.

Willard, Terry, Dr. *Mind-Body Harmony: How to Resist and Recover From Auto-Immune Diseases.* Toronto: Key Porter Books, 2003.

Printed in the United States
102051LV00002B/21/A

9 780973 986006